Diana Stobo's
Get Naked Fast!

A GUIDE TO STRIPPING AWAY THE FOODS THAT WEIGH YOU DOWN

BY DIANA STOBO

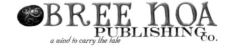

BREE NOA
PUBLISHING Co.
a wind to carry the tale

Published by Bree Noa Publishing Company
P.O. Box 204, West Linn, Oregon 97068
Email: Info@BreeNoa.com Phone: (503) 655-2386

ISBN 978-0-9840892-2-2

Printed and bound in the United States of America.

By Diana Stobo
35 Miller Ave, #188, Mill Valley, CA 94941
www.DianaStobo.com

Edited by Kristen Judy Tatroe

Book Design by Brooklyn Taylor, www.brooktown.com

Diana photographed by Allan Rosenburg and Gregg Marks

Food photographed by Diana Stobo

Photo on p. 29 courtesy of Celtic Sea Salt® Brand.

Trademarks, images, and products of Rising Tide Sea Vegetables are the property of Rising Tide Sea Vegetables.

Food For Life® and Ezekiel 4:9® are registered trademarks of Food for Life Baking Co., Inc. in the United States and other countries.

Dedication

As long as I can remember, people have come to me with food questions: How did you make that dessert? What did you dress the salad with? What should I buy when I go grocery shopping? What should I make for dinner? I've always enjoyed the questions and the teaching process. I found the inspiration for my own interests, motivation for more knowledge, and the drive to experience new avenues for the art of food through others. Over the years I have been urged, enticed, encouraged, and supported to create something tangible for others to read and refer to when they need some hand-holding in the kitchen. As time passed, my health became my primary focus. I concentrated less on "yummy" food and more on nutritional food. A natural transition occurred with the information I had to offer and I was no longer the quintessential "foodie." I became the nutritionist, the healer, and the go-to person when someone needed to make a dietary change in their life. Suddenly the nudges to write a book turned to insistence, and here we are!

I dedicate this book to the people in my life who I have inspired toward better health, good living, and "yummy" eats. Nothing gives me more joy than knowing people thirst and hunger for the knowledge to transform their lives. I thank each of you for the commitment you have to yourself, the nourishment you are providing your body and mind, and the courage it takes to Get Naked in this world today.

Strip away the foods weighing you down, feel sexier and energized, walk with confidence, look younger, live longer, and **experience the real you!**

Naked Transformations

"As I was fast approaching 50 at the beginning of the year, I decided I was going to make changes that would have a major impact on my health. I thought I was eating nutritious meals, taking my vitamins, getting in my workouts, but the truth of the matter was that most of my food didn't satisfy me anymore.

Diana's approach to food is just what I needed. She is a force of nature who has reimagined how healthy food should be. With ingredients that pack so much nutrition, **you quickly realize you're feeling and looking better without the sense that you're missing out,** and the big difference is the taste. She has such a palette for great tasting food that gives you the biggest bang for your hard-earned buck, and she never stops coming up with ways to make even the simplest snack taste like something new and different." —*Lisa C.*

. . . .

"I was already a pretty healthy eater, but my weakness was breakfast! In the morning, I loved a fried egg cooked in butter, served on top of a piece of toast generously spread with even more butter, sometimes with a slice of cheese. Once I met Diana, my whole life shifted as I began removing the six No's from my diet: wheat, dairy, meat, sugar, alcohol, and caffeine. But now what was I going to eat for breakfast? Fortunately, Diana introduced me to green drinks first thing in the morning and that boosted my clarity, energy, and vitality immediately. Then, I began making her ALT wrap for a mid-morning snack, which was delicious and substantial and would carry me through to lunch. After four months, **I've lost ten pounds while eating as much as I've wanted!** This was the stuck ten pounds that hasn't budged for two years no matter how much I exercised! Almost overnight, my body slimmed down in a totally natural, healthy way that has made me excited to get dressed again." — *Mara F.*

"I hope you can hear in the tone in my voice, the boundless energy and enthusiasm that I'm feeling with every breath that I take. It has everything to do with this diet that I am on. I don't even call it a diet—I call it my raw lifestyle. It is so amazing, I woke up this morning at 5 a.m. to go on a jog with a friend who biked next to me. It was awesome. **I feel great.** *Since going raw, I have more energy; sleep better, and even lost eight percent of my body weight*…all in less than five weeks. Through it all, Diana has been an amazing source of inspiration, information, and ongoing motivation. I cannot thank Diana enough or speak highly enough of her as **the benefits I've experienced in such a short time are incredible.** Thanks, Diana." — *Dave L.*

. . . .

"Diana Stobo has changed my life significantly. The truth is that I am in excellent shape. I enjoy endurance cycling events both on- and off-road, which leads to extremely high caloric requirements as well as deficits for recovery. Before I met Diana, I thought I had the master plan for nutrition. I studied it, lived it, and tested it.

With Diana's guidance I bridged the gap from one who thought he ate really well, to someone who truly did. With a few small tweaks of the menu, a lifestyle change took place. Not a diet, but a way to live. I am faster, recover more rapidly, sleep even better, and awaken more refreshed. From within, **my body has changed and thus the mind and spirit—transformed in a way to a place I was unaware could exist.**

One day I asked Diana about her motivation with her business, and her reply was 'to change people's lives for the better through food and love.' Well, it's true and I am so blessed to have met such a woman who embodies her qualities, and thankful that she is enlightening the rest of us." — *Benjamin B.*

Contents

Introduction

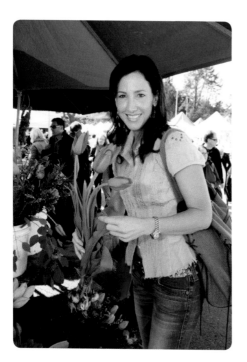

What you are about to encounter in *Get Naked Fast!* is not a diet in and of itself, but rather a way of changing your lifestyle so that you will still enjoy the wonderful sensations of amazing foods while cleaning your body, your organs, and your mind. I'll bet you've picked up this book because you care about your health. I care about your health too, and I know you're ready to transform your inner landscape as well as your outer appearance. I spent years struggling with body image, health, and the addictive food cycle. Then I came across a light and simple plan for diet and lifestyle, which I call Naked Nourishment. Once I made the commitment to change, I never looked back. If someone had told me that just cutting out a few things from my diet would have freed me from the endless cycle of worry and discontent, I would have done it eons ago. The transition to good health doesn't need to be an all-encompassing leap, but can be taken one step at a time—a gradual, thoughtful change that is made each day for yourself. Every choice, no matter how small, will have a huge impact on your overall health and beauty.

There is so much conflicting information available on nutrition—from the Internet to magazines to books—and it can be overwhelming for even the most educated person. Oftentimes we end up paralyzed, unable to move forward, only staying with what's familiar for fear of taking the wrong steps, or the information doesn't add up and can prove too difficult to assimilate. This is why my philosophy on lifestyle is as practical and simple as it gets. I keep the science to a minimum, and trust that the proof is in the pudding. There are no "shoulds" or "should-nots" in my eyes, as I believe that life is fun and we can enjoy every minute. There is no reason to be held prisoner by our diets. As long as we stay within reasonable guidelines and know the No's, we may enjoy all the flavors that nature has to offer.

Getting Naked means stripping down and simplifying the nourishment that you put in your body. I use the term Naked instead of Raw because we are often set up for failure if we strictly limit ourselves to just one thing.

Naked includes a high percentage of the Raw food diet, plus many other options for greater flexibility. If I persuade you in the beginning to exclusively try an all Raw diet, there will inevitably come a time when you are craving something familiar and cooked and feel that you are not allowed to enjoy it. But, since I believe in enjoying everything that goes into one's body, there is no room for guilt or judgment when feeding yourself. There may be times when you will feel perplexed, not knowing what to eat, and then succumb to what's available and feel as if you've fallen short of your commitment. Be as forgiving to yourself as your body will be when you quickly return to your Naked Nourishment lifestyle. You should offer yourself praise for taking the first steps to good health.

Among the many testimonials that have come in over the years from people who have followed my lifestyle plan, the most common remarks have been about one's overall state of well-being. One such person told me, "I never thought I was in poor health, but now I feel amazing, better than ever, larger than life." Another common remark is the need for less sleep, and an evenness of energy throughout the day: "I am living on five hours of sleep a night, and I wake up refreshed and excited about my day." The biggest plus about getting Naked is that you will no longer crave the foods that you were once addicted to. In fact, I hear these types of statements quite often, and they are the ones that please me most as I feel we all tend to overeat: "I have more time to do other things—I just don't think about food as much," or "I can't eat that much anymore, and my weight is exactly where I like it," or "I don't like the feeling of being full; it slows me down."

All the benefits of getting Naked will reveal themselves almost immediately. By taking things one step at a time and allowing your system to gently detox, you'll gradually wean yourself from harmful foods that keep you weighed down. You won't have to step on the scale anymore or be frustrated by the lack of results, as they will become apparent within the first few days. Your beautiful body will no longer need to struggle for balance and survival, and will begin to take full advantage of the raw energy readily available by the live, rejuvenating nourishment entering it. You will look more rested and relaxed, you will begin to effortlessly shed unwanted weight that resulted from toxic overload, your skin will brighten and smooth, and your eyes will sparkle with the inner vibrancy of your true nature. Once you begin the Naked Nourishment lifestyle, your body will begin to feel like it has gone on a vacation, and will naturally take on a glow of health, vibrance, and beauty.

The "Know No's" List

These are not restrictions, but simply facts to increase your awareness when you're eating these foods.

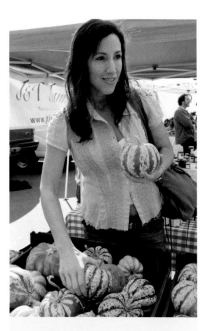

NO DAIRY:

Naturally high in protein casein and fat, dairy is hard for humans to digest. Many allergic reactions are triggered in dairy eaters and milk drinkers because humans do not produce the enzyme lactase, which is needed to break down lactose in milk. Cow's milk can cause allergic responses such as asthma, earaches, runny nose, skin rash, lethargy, and irritability. The protein casein in all milk—be it cow, goat, or human milk—releases an opiate called casomorphins during digestion. Yes, break apart the name and you end up with casein-morphine. Morphine is, of course, highly addictive and used for its calming effect. Casomorphins act as a drug in the system, similar to a morphine painkiller. (Unlike cow's milk, human milk has a small percentage of casein and high percentage of whey, so all of you mothers please don't worry—we are still giving our babies love and nutrients through our human milk.) Casein is amplified and concentrated when milk turns to cheese, increasing its opiate effects and addictive qualities. Most dairy products remain undigested in the intestines, sticking like glue to the intestinal walls, causing gas, bloating, and constipation. That creamy goodness we can't get enough of sits undigested in our intestines, creating mucous and bacteria, which are the optimum fertilizers for illness and disease.

Strip away the foods that weigh you down

- ✗ *No Dairy*
- ✗ *No Wheat*
- ✗ *No Sugar*
- ✗ *No Meat*
- ✗ *No Caffeine*
- ✗ *No Alcohol*

NO WHEAT:

Often grown with chemical fertilizers, processed with preservatives, and loaded with sugar, wheat can cause severe allergic reactions, celiac disease being just one example. Wheat contains high levels of gluten and, when consumed, this "gums up" the stomach and doesn't let other food pass, creating a rotting, putrefied environment in your intestinal tract. Processed wheat products, like breads and pastas, are the go-to food when one needs a carbohydrate fill, but it's not just the carbohydrate you're eating. Processed wheat has a high sugar content; this increases the insulin level and quickly spikes the blood sugar, making it one of the most addictive foods. Most wheat breads contain high levels of yeast, the ingredient that makes bread rise and also acts as a breeding ground for candida. Candida is an overgrowth of yeast in the human system that spreads into organ cells and tissues and causes a myriad of infections and diseases. Most grains today are processed to such a degree there is no nutritional value left. Products made from these overly processed grains simply do not provide any nutritional value and ultimately (to put it bluntly) make you fat. However, sprouted grains such as spelt, amaranth, buckwheat, millet, oats, and even wheat produce a living, nutrient-dense food. Germinating grains and seeds increases their nutrient level, digestibility, and enzymatic activity.

NO SUGAR:

Tastes sweet, smells sweet, and makes you think happy thoughts at the chance of eating it, but inside our bodies, sugar becomes a toxin. The buzz we get from eating sugar is actually our body burning excess energy to fight the poison out of our system, hence the sugar crash. Sugar causes opiates to be released within the brain, giving you an instant feel-good sensation, which in turn causes an addiction.. Sugar is a high glycemic sweetener and a breeding ground for cancer cells, is the main cause of diabetes, and accelerates the aging process. Sugar and the sugar found in processed wheat products have also been linked to ADHD, depression, and obesity.

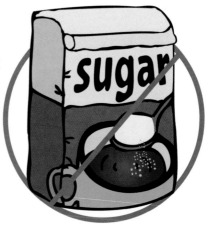

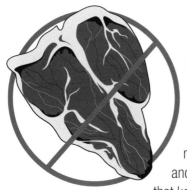

NO MEAT:

Many people are hooked on meat, and most people would balk at the idea of giving it up. What they don't realize is that meat is a leading cause of heart disease, cancer, diabetes, and other health problems. The "Holy Grail" of the American diet also takes more energy and protein to digest than you get from it. Meat proteins release opiates and spark the release of insulin. The high fat content of meat has an addictive quality that keeps you coming back for more, even if you switch to just white meat or fish. Meat nestles snugly in the digestive tract, creates inflammation in the tissues, and taxes the kidneys. Because meat moves slowly through the digestive system, it releases uric acid into the bloodstream, muscles, and tissue, causing an over-acidic breeding ground for infection and disease. Uric acid is the number one cause of gout, otherwise known as "rich man's disease," which plagues a large percentage of our meat-eating nation. The good news is once you stop eating meat for a few weeks, you will stop craving it.

NO CAFFEINE:

What goes up must come down. The burst of energy you get from caffeine is actually your body screaming "Poison!" as it rushes to counteract the toxin. Caffeine is a quick-fix pleasure with a huge downside as it overworks the adrenal glands and spikes blood sugar, leaving you anxious and restless. It reduces absorption of iron and zinc by up to 50%, which ultimately taxes your immune system. Caffeine is very acidic to the body and pulls calcium from the bones to neutralize the acids; this leaves you in a chronic state of calcium deficiency which can eventually result in osteoporosis.

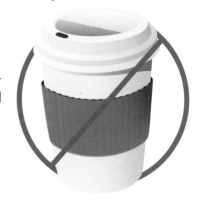

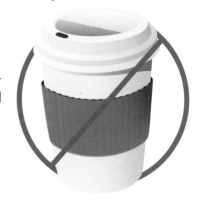

NO ALCOHOL:

It gives us a false sense of lightness, sexiness, divine energy, and joy, but really alcohol exhausts our energy, depletes our vitamins and minerals, and leads to dehydration and toxicity. What begins as a euphoric romp with "the spirits," ends in the quintessential hangover. Alcohol puts a strain on our digestive system and liver. Its depressant attributes make it highly addictive, and consuming too much can lead to degenerative cell tissue, strained organs, and ultimately obesity and fatigue. Alcohol also affects the skin by accelerating the aging process, increasing wrinkles, and causing dry skin and loss of elasticity.

The Balancing Act

The Acid/Alkaline Body

A Balanced Life begins from within as good nutrition, and reflects out into the world as joy, peace, and happiness.

Balancing your Acid/Alkaline Body

Our bodies are constantly striving for balance. What we eat and how we live can help us with this balancing act. Eating an alkaline diet with the right balance of neutral to acidic foods, along with being an all-around happy person, will help us maintain the perfect alkaline state.

How do we know if we are too acidic or too alkaline? There are signs to look for (see chart below), but testing your urine with pH litmus paper each morning may also be a helpful indicator. Litmus paper can be found online or in health food stores.

Signs of Over-Acidity in the Body

- Overweight
- Blotchy or unhealthy skin
- Discoloration of skin
- Acne
- Itchy scalp
- Chronic fatigue
- Chronic headaches
- Chronic negative thoughts
- Anxiety
- Anger
- Insomnia
- Depression
- Tense muscles
- High stress
- Extreme highs and lows throughout the day
- Addiction to coffee, alcohol, cigarettes, marijuana, any other drug (prescription or otherwise)

Signs of Over-Alkalinity in the Body

- Lethargy
- Mental spaciness
- Extreme passivity
- Cold extremities
- Lack of enthusiasm or drive

Some people weigh themselves. I check my litmus paper to see where I may be out of balance.

Signs of an Acid/Alkaline Balanced Body

- High energy
- Feeling balanced
- Mental clarity
- Clear skin
- Bright eyes
- Perfect weight for body type
- Positive thoughts
- Calm
- Loving
- Inspiring

How to Create Alkalinity

- Foods rich in alkaline minerals
- Green juice
- Alkaline water
- Love
- Passion
- Sex
- Friendship
- Intimacy
- Skipping
- Dancing
- Laughter
- Joy
- Algae
- Chlorophyll
- Being in nature
- Long walks
- Breathing deeply

How to Create Acidity

- Foods rich in acidic minerals
- Worry
- Stress
- Fear
- Anger
- Sugar
- Wheat
- Alcohol
- Caffeine
- Meat
- Dairy
- Watching too much television
- No exercise
- Too much time in front of the computer
- Prescription drugs
- Smoking
- Short, shallow breathing

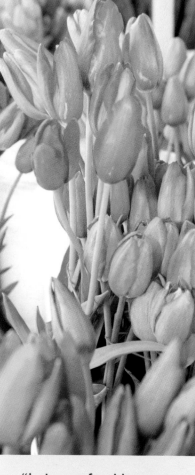

"Let your food be your medicine, and your medicine be your food."
~ *Hippocrates*

Disease cannot live in an alkaline environment.

Ranked Food Chart: Alkaline To Acidic

EXTREMELY ALKALINE

Lemons, Watermelon

ALKALINE FORMING

Cantaloupe, Cayenne, Celery, Dates, Figs, Kelp, Limes, Mango, Melons, Papaya, Parsley, Seaweeds, Seedless Grapes, Watercress, Asparagus, Fruit Juices, Grapes, Kiwifruit, Passionfruit, Pears, Pineapple, Raisins, Umeboshi Plums, Vegetable Juices

MODERATELY ALKALINE

Apples, Alfalfa Sprouts, Apricots, Avocados, Bananas, Currants, Dates, Figs, Garlic, Grapefruit, Grapes (less sweet), Guavas, Herbs, Lettuce, Nectarines, Peaches, Pears (less sweet), Peas, Pumpkins, Sea Salt, Apples (sour), Green Beans, Beets, Bell Peppers, Broccoli, Cabbage, Carob, Cauliflower, Ginger, Grapes (sour), Lettuce (pale green), Oranges, Peaches (less sweet), Peas (less sweet), Potatoes (with skin), Pumpkin (less sweet), Raspberries, Strawberries, Squash, Sweet Corn, Turnips, Apple Cider Vinegar

SLIGHTLY ALKALINE

Almonds, Jerusalem Artichokes, Brussels Sprouts, Cherries, Coconut (fresh), Cucumbers, Eggplant, Honey (raw), Leeks, Mushrooms, Okra, Olives (ripe), Onions, Pickles (homemade), Radishes, Sea Salt, Spices, Tomatoes, Brown Rice Vinegar, Chestnuts (dry, roasted), Egg Yolks, Essene Bread, Goat's Milk and Whey (raw), Mayonnaise (homemade), Olive Oil, Sesame Seeds (whole), Soy Beans (dry), Soy Cheese, Soy Milk, Sprouted Grains, Tofu, Tomatoes (less sweet), Nutritional Yeast

NEUTRAL

Butter (fresh, unsalted), Cream (fresh, raw), Cow's Milk and Whey (raw), Margarine, Oils (except olive), Yogurt (plain)

MODERATELY ACIDIC

Bananas (green), Barley (rye), Blueberries, Bran, Butter, Cereals (unrefined), Cheeses, Crackers (unrefined rye, rice, and wheat), Cranberries, Dried Beans (mung, adzuki, pinto, kidney, garbanzo), Dry Coconut, Egg Whites, Eggs Whole (cooked hard), Fructose, Goat's Milk (homogenized), Honey (pasteurized), Ketchup, Maple Syrup (unprocessed), Cow's Milk (homogenized), Molasses (unsulfured and organic), Most Nuts, Mustard, Oats (rye, organic), Olives (pickled), Pasta (whole grain), Pastries (whole grain and honey), Plums, Popcorn (with salt and/or butter), Potatoes, Prunes, Rice (basmati and brown), Seeds (pumpkin, sunflower), Soy Sauce, Wheat Bread (sprouted organic)

EXTREMELY ACIDIC

Artificial Sweeteners, Beef, Beer, Breads, Brown Sugar, Carbonated Soft Drinks, Cereals (refined), Chocolate, Cigarettes and Tobacco, Coffee, Cream of Wheat (unrefined), Custard (with white sugar), Deer, Drugs, Fish, Flour (white wheat), Fruit Juices with Sugar, Jams, Jellies, Lamb, Liquor, Maple Syrup (processed), Molasses (sulfured), Pasta (white), Pastries and Cakes from White Flour, Pickles (commercial), Pork, Poultry, Seafood, Sugar (white), Table Salt (refined and iodized), Tea (black), White Bread, White Vinegar (processed), Whole Wheat Foods, Wine, Yogurt (sweetened)

Questions about Naked Nourishment

Eating Naked or Raw foods, or foods that are not heated beyond 118 degrees, will bring a life force energy that will ultimately heal and enhance your being. Eating foods with life-enriching energy will literally transfer the wholesome force directly into your body giving you more vibrance, better health, and radiant beauty. Choosing to step away from the Standard American Diet (SAD) into something more unique is a gift that will help you gain energy, drop excess weight, think more clearly, love more deeply, and give you an overall glow.

What can I expect when I Get Naked?

For most, an immediate improvement in their overall health, quick and effortless weight loss, clearer skin, less wrinkles, an abundance of energy, lack of need for sleep, less aches and pains, and an overall youthful appearance. You will find any ailment or disease reversing dramatically and rapidly as your body begins to take on the life force energy of live food and the swift elimination of the products that are ailing you.

The reason to know the No's list?

Ultimately this is the foundation for both a healthy diet and lifestyle. Many foods could be considered raw but I would *never* eat them. Raw meat and dairy are two examples, as neither meat nor dairy is healthy to eat in the raw form. They are laden with bacteria and infection, which is why we began pasteurizing and cooking them long ago—to kill what kills us. While it is true that meat and dairy have some benefits, such as protein and calcium, there are no benefits that you cannot attain from a plant-based diet, so I believe the harm that comes to the body is much greater than any offering. If you haven't already done so, read the "Know No's" section (page 4) to learn more about what these products do to your body. Use it as a starting point to do your own research.

Why don't I just go 100% raw?

This should be an easier transition, if it is done slowly and properly. The key to success is moderation and knowing the facts. Remember, everything worthwhile takes time, including the management of your overall wellness. Each step you take toward the Naked Nourishment philosophy will immediately reveal itself physically, mentally, and emotionally through you. The body is sensible and it understands when you are attending to it. It will adapt to any healthy lifestyle changes you introduce, and it wants you to succeed and live an amazing, wholesome life. You may at any time opt for an all-raw meal, and simply use the cooked versions as backup when you desire warm food.

I eat pretty healthy. How do I begin to Get Naked?

The first step is to "clean house." We'll go into more detail in The Naked Pantry Makeover section, but for now take a look inside your refrigerator and pantry and remove all processed or manufactured foods. Trash those products and promise yourself never to spend your hard-earned money on them again.

The second step is stop believing everything you hear about the body's need for calcium, protein, carbohydrates, and fats. Know that most of the information medical professionals give is driven by the media and supported by pharmaceutical companies and farmers. Their information will only cause you to second-guess yourself and the process of regaining health, and ultimately sabotage your choice to eat healthy. You are your best doctor, so just listen to yourself. Your body will always let you know what it needs.

The third is to avoid the "Know No's" (no dairy, no wheat, no sugar, no meat, no alcohol, and no caffeine) and begin an intake of live plant foods: vegetables, fruits, nuts, and sprouted grains. The key to a Naked Nourishment lifestyle is versatility and creativity.

Finally, ask yourself three simple questions before purchasing any foods:

"Is it healthy or not healthy for my body?"
We all have a natural sensibility about what our body truly likes, desires, and needs in order to thrive. We generally don't listen to that innate voice, but take an extra minute to ask yourself if your body really wants that food. If you have to think about it, it's probably not healthy for you.

"Is it raw (processed at or under 118 degrees)?"
Besides the natural raw and organic produce that you may consume at anytime, ask yourself about other questionable products before you eat them. Find out if they were heated or processed at a high heat, which leaves them with virtually little nutritional value.

"Has the food been processed?"
It's safe to say that anything that has a long shelf life has been processed, preserved, tampered with, or modified in some way that it no longer resembles any sense of real food. Don't even bother with it. It will only serve you if you would like to see it stored on the shelves of your hips or waist.

What percentage of live raw food should I consume to start?

Start by eating 50% of raw foods. You may be surprised at how little fresh food you were putting into your body before you began to Get Naked. This can be quickly accomplished by choosing drinks and smoothies made of fresh fruits and vegetables for breakfast and snacks. They will fill you up, nourish you, and guarantee your 50% goal. Ultimately, a 70-80% diet of pure live raw food will bring you a lean and healthy life of joy, energy, and vitality.

What are the essentials I must have in my home in order to get started?

It's hard to say how much of a transition this will be for you, since I don't know what your pantry looks like. I try not to make assumptions, but a household usually has a decent blender and food processor. That's a good start! As you become more committed to your lifestyle, your needs may change. Check out the Naked Necessities section (page 31) for more equipment choices.

As for food items, simple is best. Since you are about to clean out your pantry of old processed foods that will no longer feed you, what do you place in your pantry instead? Check out the substitution list for items that will feed and nourish you in a moment's notice. Most importantly, though, buy live plant food. This means vegetables and fruits of your choosing, and fresh herbs and sprouts as well.

How important is eating organic if I am eating mostly raw foods?

Always think organic when buying your food. The word "organic" has frightened us in the past, as we saw it as something unique that we couldn't find in our supermarkets, but "organic" just means natural, free of pesticides, herbicides, and fungicides, and hopefully grown in a mineral rich soil. Organic produce need not be washed, especially if grown at home or purchased at a farmers market. If at any time you are unable to find organic produce, wash your fruits and vegetables carefully with a food grade hydrogen peroxide that will strip the chemicals from the plant so that you will not ingest them. Certain foods—such as avocados, bananas, and coconuts—are more protected from the chemicals as they have a thicker skin, but is debatable how much of the chemical penetrates the food. Be aware that washing is not a long-term solution as non-organic foods will still be lower in mineral content due to the conditions of the soil in which they're grown. This is an important consideration since minerals are the key component to gaining health, vibrancy, and beauty.

I'm used to eggs, toast, or cereal for breakfast. What should I eat that won't take too long to make?

Start your day off with an energy boost, not something that will weigh you down. Think smoothies! Everybody loves smoothies, but we seem to have a mental block against considering them as a meal since many people categorize them in the "drink" department. Green smoothies are a great way to consume your Naked greens for the day. Ultimately, you should consume two full bunches of greens each day. A mental measure I use to evaluate my intake is what you would buy in the market: a bunch of spinach, a bunch of chard, a bunch of lettuce. If you're thinking "salad," it might seem like a chore to consume that many greens, but transforming them into a yummy smoothie might change your mind. Blending your daily Naked greens into a drink along with a fruit or fresh pressed juice will help the vitamins and minerals absorb quickly and make it an enjoyable breakfast to wake up to. (See Recipes for great smoothie ideas.)

I'm addicted to coffee—I can't start my day without it. What should I do?

This is the most common question, and I give the same answer every time: enjoy your coffee. If this is the one vice you have while alleviating all the other toxins from your body, then have your 'cup of joe' and enjoy it. But try having just one cup, and if the mood strikes again in the middle of the day, go for a green juice or smoothie instead. You will find the boost you get from live food is far greater than that of caffeine. I also suggest trying an organic low acid coffee and switching from cream to almond cream, and sugar to stevia or agave. In the end, I think moderation is a key to success.

What happens when I'm hungry?

It's simple: you eat. Naked Nourishment should never be considered a diet, but a lifestyle. It's a choice to take your health into your own hands. If losing weight is your goal, you will never have to count calories again. Eat as much as you want. The more greens and Naked live foods you put in your body, the stronger foundation you are building for your health. You will find that if your choices remain in the live foods, specifically greens, you will ultimately eat less. You will dissolve all cravings, and find that your relationship with food has taken a turn. You will no longer be dependent on emotional quick-fix eats; you will discover that food becomes a part of your medicinal, nutritional landscape, and you will derive great pleasure from simple, natural, and pure foods.

What can I snack on?

If you are thinking outside of fresh produce (cherry tomatoes, avocados, carrots, apples, oranges, etc.) and are looking for something that fulfills the comfort need or sweet cravings, then go for Naked, raw nuts or raw granolas. You can even snack on a homemade trail mix—there are many options for those 'tween' hunger pangs. Check out recipe ideas later on, in the Recipe section, or check out my website (www.DianaStobo.com) for some recipe tips to engage in a more versatile snack menu.

What about supplements?

I like to think of the supplements I take as Superfoods. The few things that I adhere to each day are: chewing on chlorella tablets, which have an abundance of plant-based protein; E3Live™, which is a blue-green algae; my digestive enzymes, of course; and an array of other whole food nutritional boosts. It's best to clean out your system before adding any more confusion. Someone told me that you have to break down the system first before you can rebuild it, so for now let's just start by Getting Naked!

Can you give me a sample menu and help me plan my day?

Sample Menu

6 a.m. – 9 a.m.	Breakfast	Smoothie, juice, or drink
9 a.m. – 12 p.m.	Mid-morning	Fruit, grain cereal, or smoothie
12 p.m. – 3 p.m.	Lunch	Salad, soup, or wrap
3 p.m. – 6 p.m.	Mid-afternoon	Smoothie or green juice
6 p.m. – 9 p.m.	Dinner	Salad, soup, or grain bowl
9 p.m. – 12 a.m.	Evening	Hot tea or sweet snack

If you work in an office, you'll need to plan for mid-morning, lunch, and mid-afternoon items. You could also easily adjust your mid-afternoon smoothie to a raw snack or raw trail mix.

I like having a glass of wine before dinner. Is that still okay?

I have the same response to wine as I have for coffee: have a glass of wine. Be cognizant of why you are drinking and how much you are drinking. Coffee and wine are stimulants and depressants, but they also bring a little spice to life. The key in health is to find balance. If you are not finding joy in your healing process, then you are not healing. So, you get to choose your vice. Wine is a fermented food and therefore raw, but while it may have some health benefits, I say drink freshly made grape juice instead. Knowing that alcohol is acidic to your cellular structure, I would alleviate hard alcohol and limit wine in your Naked Nourishment lifestyle. However, if it makes you happy, choose organic sulfite-free wines. Your happiness is a much more powerful healing tool.

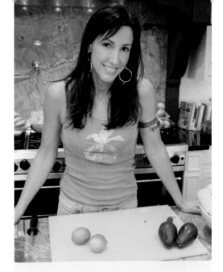

If you are not finding joy in your healing process, then you are not healing.

I love to eat out. What do you think of dining out?

Dining out can be such a lovely social experience, and I would never suggest it be overlooked. Eating out for the mere pleasure of food is another wonderful experience. If the social aspect is what you are asking about, then my simple suggestion would be to fill yourself with a highly nutritious meal before you go out. Order a salad or something light to maintain the joy of the occasion. If you are asking about craving a culinary experience, then my answer is go and enjoy every bite; great culinary art is something nobody should miss. This is your life, and you get to choose how quickly you wish to Get Naked. If you are merely craving fast food, a quick fix, something naughty in your body, perhaps you should think twice. The foods served in chain restaurants and fast food joints are laden with bad salts and cooked oils—it's no wonder they taste so good! But there is very little nutritional value, and ultimately your body will let you know how it feels after you eat it.

I get low blood sugar. Are you sure I'll be okay on a raw food diet?

As your body detoxifies, your blood sugar will begin to level out and you will no longer experience blood sugar lows. One of the most noticeable changes when you introduce more raw plant food into your diet is the amount of food you will need. You will discover that you automatically adjust to a different pace or interval of eating. You may have been used to eating three large meals, but will find you adjust to consuming less food more often throughout the day. On a raw diet, your body will feel full and nourished more quickly as you are receiving more nutrients per mouthful. This shift is not only easier on your digestive tract, but will ultimately speed up your metabolism as your body is working more efficiently. Listen to your body—it will let you know what it needs.

Will I get enough protein without meat?

The greatest misconception is that we need more protein. There is more than enough protein in a multiple, plant-based diet. The truth is the protein from meat is so hard to digest and process through the human digestive tract, it ends up leaving you at a deficit for muscle-building proteins. In a Naked Nourishment lifestyle, you can trust you're getting enough proteins from produce and nuts.

Protein Calories in Food

Vegetables

Alfalfa sprouts	40%
Artichoke	29%
Asparagus	25%
Bamboo shoots	26%
Beet greens	22%
Broccoli	49%
Brussels sprouts	49%
Cabbage, Chinese	12%
Cabbage, red	20%
Cauliflower	27%
Celery	10%
Chard, Swiss	24%
Chives	18%
Collards (leaves)	48%
Collards (stems)	36%
Cress	26%
Cucumber	10%
Dandelion greens	27%
Eggplant	12%
Fennel	28%
Garlic	20%
Kale (leaves)	60%
Leek	22%
Lettuce, Boston	12%
Lettuce, green-leaf	42%
Lettuce, iceberg	27%
Lettuce, loose-leaf	13%
Mustard greens	22%
Okra	24%
Onion (green)	15%
Parsley	36%
Pepper, green	12%
Pepper, red	14%
Pepper, red hot	13%
Radish	10%
Rhubarb	11%
Seaweed, dulse	25%
Spinach	49%
Turnip greens	30%
Watercress	22%
Wheat grass	25%
Zucchini	26%

Fruits

Avocado (California)	22%
Avocado (Florida)	15%
Grapefruit, sour	5%
Lemon	13%
Lemon juice	5%
Tomato, green	12%
Tomato, red	18%

Legumes

Chickpea	25%
Lentil	30%
Lima bean, fresh	9%
Mung sprouts	38%
Navy bean	26%
Pea, green fresh	6%
Red bean, fresh	9%
Soybean, dried	34%
Soybean, fresh	11%
Soybean sprouts	6%

Nuts and Seeds

Brazil Nut	14%
Filbert	13%
Pumpkin seed	29%
Sesame seed	19%
Sunflower seed	24%
Sunflower seed, sprouted	33%

Grains

Barley	10%
Millet	10%
Rice, brown	8%
Wheat	17%
Wheat bran	16%

Will I get enough calcium without dairy?

The calcium from dairy cannot be assimilated into our bodies. We do not produce the proper enzymes to digest dairy products, therefore it becomes stagnate and acidic in our system. Calcium is in fact leached from our bones in order to balance dairy's acidic nature. In a Naked Nourishment lifestyle, you will get enough easily digestible calcium from a plant-based diet.

Calcium in Food

Vegetables

Artichoke......................51 mg
Asparagus....................23 mg
Bamboo shoot..............13 mg
Beet greens.................119 mg
Broccoli.......................103 mg
Brussels sprout.............36 mg
Cabbage, Chinese.........43 mg
Cabbage, red................42 mg
Cauliflower...................25 mg
Celery.........................39 mg
Chard, Swiss................88 mg
Chives.........................69 mg
Collards (leaves)..........250 mg
Collards (stems)..........203 mg
Cress..........................81 mg
Cucumber....................25 mg
Dandelion greens........187 mg
Eggplant......................12 mg
Fennel........................100 mg
Garlic..........................29 mg
Kale (leaves)...............249 mg
Kale (stem).................179 mg
Leek............................52 mg
Lettuce, Boston.............35 mg
Lettuce, iceberg............20 mg
Lettuce, loose-leaf........68 mg
Mustard greens..........183 mg
Okra............................92 mg
Onion (green)................51 mg
Parsley.......................203 mg
Pepper, green.................9 mg
Pepper, red...................13 mg
Pepper, red hot...........130 mg
Radish.........................30 mg
Rhubarb.......................96 mg
Seaweed, agar............567 mg
Seaweed, dulse..........296 mg
Spinach........................93 mg
Turnip greens.............246 mg
Watercress.................151 mg

Fruits

Avocado (California)......10 mg
Avocado (Florida)..........10 mg
Grapefruit, sour.............16 mg
Lemon juice....................7 mg
Tomato, green..............13 mg
Tomato, red..................13 mg

Legumes

Chickpea.....................150 mg
Lentil, dried..................79 mg
Lima bean, fresh...........52 mg
Mung sprouts..............118 mg
Pea, green fresh...........26 mg
Red bean, dried..........110 mg
Soybean, dried............226 mg
Soybean, fresh.............67 mg
Soybean, sprouts..........48 mg

Nuts and Seeds

Almond.......................234 mg
Brazil nut....................186 mg
Filbert........................209 mg
Pumpkin seed...............51 mg
Sesame seed...........1,160 mg
Sunflower seed...........120 mg

Grains

Barley.........................34 mg
Millet..........................20 mg
Rice, brown.................32 mg
Wheat.........................46 mg
Wheat bran................119 mg

The Naked Pantry Makeover

Strip away the foods that hold you hostage… because it feels so good.

What's in your kitchen now? Take a look around, and start pulling out the things that will no longer serve you. Don't get attached to the box of granola bars that has been sitting there waiting for a rainy day. Think about how long they've been there and how much longer they will last; the amount of preservatives holding them together will only cause discomfort in your body. If you are attached to them, place them in a box in the garage in case there really is some grand disaster and you are in fear of starving. For now, though, you are alive and well and ready to Get Naked! This is it, the way you have always wanted to live, stripped of the foods that hold you hostage. This section is a makeover for your pantry, refrigerator, and cupboards. It will also serve as a shopping list enabling you to pull together healthful meals in just moments.

Farmers markets are a great place to find some of these essentials. It is a place where real food is sold directly from the fields or farmers' kitchens, fully alive and completely nourishing. Try to visit your local farmers market for the freshest ingredients and the freshest lifestyle. Buying locally will help sustain our lifestyle as well as our earth.

Coconuts

Young Thai coconuts are a must in my home. The water in a coconut has the highest level of electrolytes of any plant food. They will perk up any wilted flower on a hot summer day. They are available in Asian markets as well as health food stores. Go to www.DianaStobo.com to watch my video on how to break open a coconut.

Fresh Fruits

Fresh fruits are a great way to get a sweet treat and an energy pick-me-up. If you are healing and want to cleanse on a deep level, minimize or eliminate your fruit intake. But for a healthy diet, fruit will aid you in pleasing ways. Low glycemic fruits are all citrus: grapefruits, oranges, limes, and lemons. Berries such as raspberries, strawberries, blackberries, blueberries, and even huckleberries are high in vitamin C and are great for the skin. Açai berries are sweeping the nation with their important antioxidants. Since they are hard to find fresh or dried, try a frozen version and add them to your smoothie, but don't buy into the hype and limit yourself to açai berries—it's important to diversify.

Fresh Herbs

Fresh herbs are another item you can't do without. I tend to always have parsley, cilantro, and mint on hand, but dill, basil, and other fresh herbs come and go depending on what's being prepared.

Good Fats

There are lots of oils—good oils—that fall into this category. Organic cold pressed olive oils are wonderful for your body. Bariani brand is excellent, but note that some cold pressed olive oils may turn bitter when blended. Pumpkin seed oil is rich and delicious; I love this blended with fresh citrus for a light salad dressing. Hemp seed oil can be a little heavy tasting, but it's nice with other strong flavors for added nutrition. Flax oil, which is mild and delicious, is good for all uses, and I love it in smoothies. My favorite, though, is Udo's Choice™ Oil Blend. When my skin is feeling dry, I add a tablespoon in my morning smoothie to nourish my skin from the inside out. It also thickens the smoothie to a whole other level. Essential Balance®, another nice blended oil, contains a hint of borage oil.

Grains

I try not to go too crazy with the starches, but I always have buckwheat groats, although they're really a seed. Groats are simply the hulled grain. Examples of hearty, non-glutenous grains are oat groats, quinoa, amaranth, rye, and winter wheat berries. At times, I will buy spelt, millet, and kamut for variation. However, I keep brown rice to a minimum, as it's more glutenous than the other grains.

Legumes

I am into garbanzo beans (also known as chickpeas), mung beans, lentils, peas, and adzuki beans for sprouting. They are great on salads, and when making a hummus nothing beats the flavor or nutrients of sprouted chickpeas. Other legumes to consider are kidney beans, black-eyed peas, pinto beans, and black beans. Never buy canned as the canning process makes the legumes acidic to the body. Check your local farmers market. I just discovered fresh raw chickpeas, and they make the most outrageous hummus.

Milks

It's always smart to have pre-made milk on hand. Pacific Natural Foods makes almond milk, hazelnut milk, and an array of other milks. My favorites are still the freshly-made milks from raw soaked nuts, but in a pinch, pre-made milk is fine. For a quick nut milkshake, check out the Recipes section.

Nuts

Raw nuts are a must in your pantry. I stock raw nut butters for ease and convenience—they're great for instant nut milks, spreads, and sauces. I generally have a large supply of raw almonds so I can prepare a batch of almond milk every four days. It's super easy, delicious, and more convenient than running to the store for a half-gallon of milk. I also stock Brazil nuts, pecans, macadamia nuts, pine nuts, walnuts, hazelnuts, and cashews. Each nut has its own character, set of nutrients, and unique flavors. They are great for desserts, cheeses, pâtes, nut milks, cookies, and just eating raw.

Produce

The beauty about produce is that it's beautifying. Anything you choose will benefit and nourish you. It's best to select what's local, organic, and in season for the freshest, most nourishing and mineralizing food. I try to pick up fresh produce a couple times a week. I always have an array of green produce on hand: I use chard and lettuce to wrap other veggies for a quick raw sandwich. Avocados are a must, as they are often used as the "meat" of my wraps. It seems color is key to variety, so try red bell peppers, carrots, beets, radishes, mushrooms, zucchini, celery, cucumber, spinach, cabbage, kale, and tomatoes. These are just a few essentials. I also dabble in roots for a more hearty meal, including such items as celeriac (celery root), burdock root, sun chokes, basically things which we don't see in everyday food preparation but that offer great nutrients and fabulous taste.

Sea Veggies

These should be considered a staple, as nothing will mineralize the body quicker. Since we are a sushi-loving nation, most of us are familiar with nori sheets. Just take the white rice and fish out of the equation and roll away! Wrap anything green between these sheets to make a delicious roll: avocado, baby greens, carrots, cucumber—the list goes on and on. I also have dulse in whole form as well as flakes—it's great as a sprinkle on salads and soups as well as equally good to nibble on instead of chips. I like wakame as well. It's nice to throw it in a broth for slow cooking, as it adds a nice salty mineralized character. These are just my staples. There are other sea vegetables that have great flavors, so don't be afraid to explore.

Seeds

Seeds are generally inexpensive and packed full of vitamins and protein. These can also be made into milks, pâtes, or cheeses, but they are equally delicious just raw. In my pantry are sunflower seeds, sesame seeds, hemp seeds, pumpkin seeds, flax seeds, and chia seeds.

Sprouted Breads and Tortillas

These are my go-to splurge when I'm feeling that need to indulge a little. I always have sprouted grain tortillas, sprouted corn tortillas, and spelt tortillas on hand. I have pita pockets, Ezekiel 4:9® Srouted Whole Grain English Muffins, and when I need a little sweetness, Fruit & Nut Manna Bread® in the freezer. A spoonful of pecan butter with a date on top will take care of any cravings and keep me from straying toward the "old ways."

Sweeteners

Dried fruits such as dates, figs, raisins, and cranberries are the best way to get sweetness into a recipe. Currants are a nice surprise mixed with tomatoes, and don't forget the ever powerful Goji berry which I consume in quantity as I mix them in with my nut milks. A good alternative to sugar is raw blue agave, a light syrup that sweetens with a low glycemic index. Raw wild honey or bee propolis are both highly mineralized sweeteners, and maple syrup, although not raw, provides sweet satisfaction without the effects of processed sugars.

Naked Substitutions

As with any change in life, it's better to start slow and make steady progress to ensure you can sustain the improvements. It often takes several trials to make something a habit, so just keep trying and you'll succeed. Integrate the new foods into your life one step at a time, and pick the simplest and most usable items to start.

When you first begin to Know the No's, you'll want a substitution that will work within your current diet. Begin by replacing your usual cow's milk with a non-dairy milk like an almond milk or a rice milk, or replacing your usual wheat bread with an Ezekiel 4:9® Organic Sprouted 100% Whole Grain Flourless Bread. This way, you can make a small change in your diet that will make a big difference to your body. Below is a substitution list with some popular brands that I have tried and really love. Feel free to explore several different options in each category to find the solution that best suits your palate.

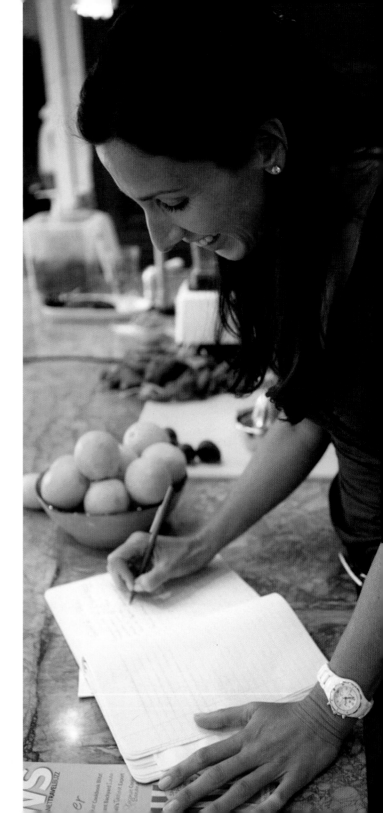

Dairy

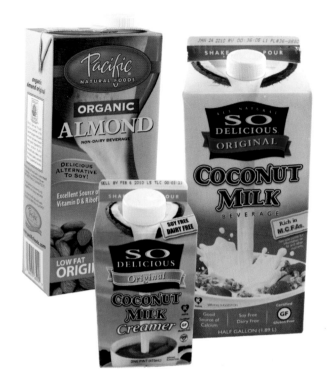

Milk and Cream

- Pacific Natural Foods: organic nut and grain non-dairy beverages
- So Delicious® Coconut Milk Beverage
- So Delicious® Coconut Milk Creamer
- Any available organic rice, nut or hemp milk

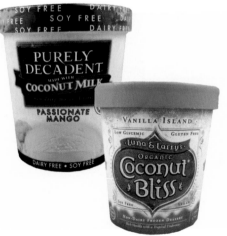

Ice Cream

- Luna & Larry's Coconut Bliss™ (certified organic non-dairy frozen dessert, coconut milk-based)
- Purely Decadent® (non-dairy frozen dessert made with coconut milk)

Butter

- Ancient Organics: Ghee (a clarified butter that is no longer in a dairy state)
- Purity Farms: Ghee
- Rejuvenative Foods: Organic Cashew Butter, Organic Walnut Butter, Organic Pecan Butter, Organic Brazil Nut Butter, Organic Hazelnut Butter, Organic Raw Almond Butter, Organic Raw Tahini
- Artisana™ Nut and Seed Butters: Raw Almond Butter, Raw Cashew Butter, Raw Macadamia Butter, Raw Pecan Butter, Raw Walnut Butter, Raw Tahini (great for quick seed and nut milks, as well as spreads and sauces)

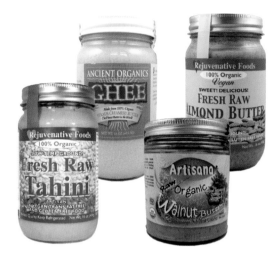

Yogurt

- Ricera®: Rice Milk Yogurt
- So Delicious® Coconut Yogurt

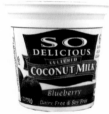
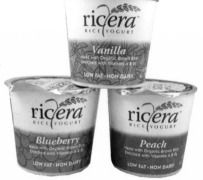

Cheese

- Eat in the Raw: Parma!™ (a nut parmesan cheese)
- Lifeway®: Helios Kefir
- Clover Organic Farms: Organic Kefir
- Nancy's® Organic Kefir

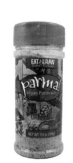
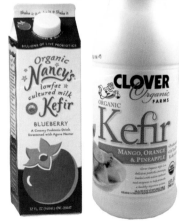

Wheat

Bread

- Ezekiel 4:9® Organic Sprouted 100% Whole Grain Flourless Bread
- Pacific Bakery: spelt breads, kamut breads, millet breads, rye breads, sprouted grain breads
- Manna Organics: Manna Bread®
- Rudi's Organic: Spelt Bread

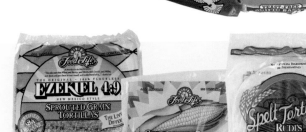

Tortillas

- Ezekiel 4:9® Sprouted Grain Tortillas and Ezekiel 4:9® Sprouted Corn Tortillas
- Rudi's Organic: Spelt Tortillas

English Muffins

- Food for Life® Organic Sprouted 100% Whole Grain & Seed English Muffins
- Rudi's Organic: Spelt English Muffins

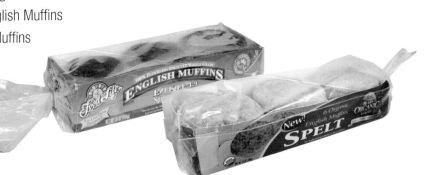

Bagels
- French Meadow Bakery™: sprouted grain bagels
- Alvarado Street Bakery: sprouted grain bagels

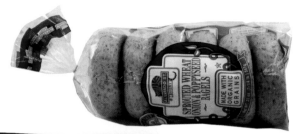

Cereals
- Kaia Foods: raw granola
- GoRaw: raw granola

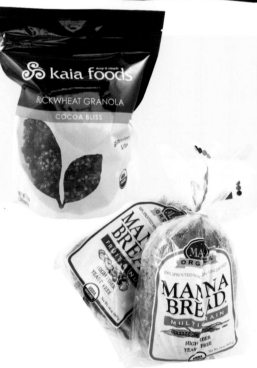

Cake Breads
- Manna Organics: Fruit & Nut Manna Bread®
  (distributed by Nature's Path Foods Inc.)

Grains
- Ancient Harvest® brand Quinoa
- Alter Eco™: Fair Trade Organic Black Quinoa,
  Red Quinoa, Pearl Quinoa

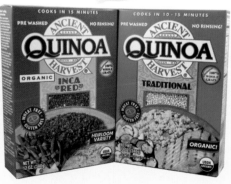

Caffeine

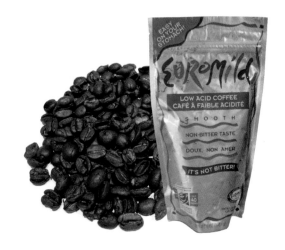

Coffee
- Euromild™: Acid Free Coffee
- Organic, fair trade coffee

Tea
- Yogi™ Tea
- Triple Leaf Tea
- Traditional Medicinals® Tea

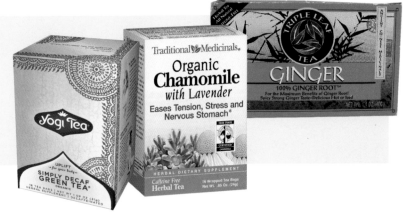

Energy Drinks
- GT's Raw Organic Kombucha
- Synergy Organic & Raw
- O.N.E.™ Coconut Water
- Amy & Brian All Natural Coconut Juice

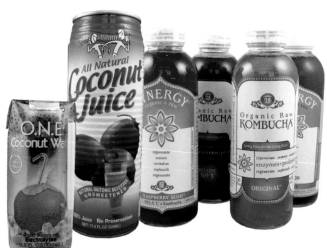

Sweeteners

Sugar

- Raw Agave Nectar
- Shady Maple Farms Maple Syrup
- Stevia leaf powder or liquid
- Alter Eco™: Organic Ground Cane Sugar
- Wholesome Sweeteners®: Organic Sucanat
- Really Raw® Honey
- Pure, organic maple syrup

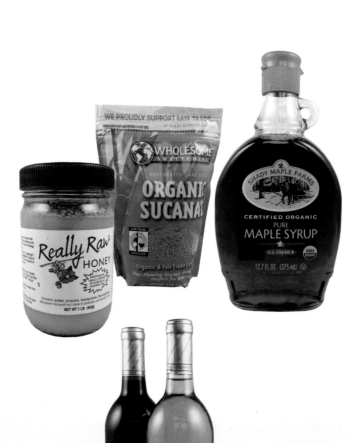

Alcohol

Wine

- Frey Vineyards (organic wine with no sulfites)

Supplements

- Essential Balance® 3-6-9 Blended Oil
- E3Live™
- Chlorella

Condiments

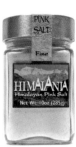
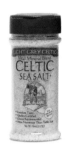
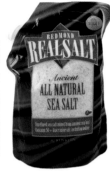

Salt
- Himalania® Himalayan Pink Crystal Salt
- Redmond: Real Salt®
- Celtic Sea Salt® Brand

Savory
- Maine Coast Sea Vegetables
- Bragg Liquid Aminos
- Ohsawa® Organic Nama® Shoyu
- Emerald Cove® Sea Vegetables
- Rising Tide Sea Vegetables

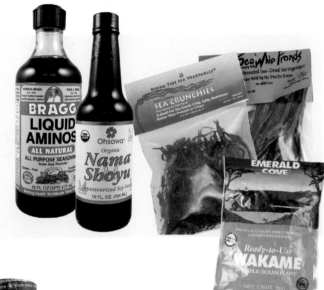

Dressing
- Follow Your Heart® Vegenaise®

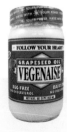

Broth
- Pacific Natural Foods

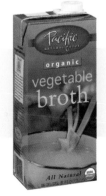

Vinegar

- Bragg Organic Apple Cider Vinegar
- Organic rice wine vinegar
- Eden® Selected Ume Plum Paste and Vinegar
- Eden® Selected Red Wine Vinegar

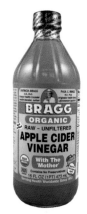

Pickles (fermented foods)

- Cultured®: Raw Sauerkraut
- Alexander Valley Gourmet: Pickles and Sauerkraut
- Bubbies®: Pickles and Sauerkraut
- Rejuvenate Foods Fresh Cultured Live Salsa

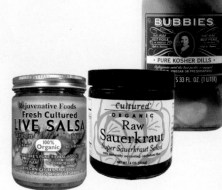

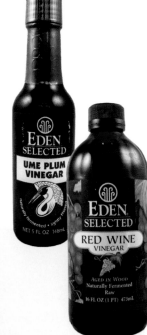

Oil

- Bariani: Olive Oil (stone crushed, cold pressed)
- Nutiva®: Hemp Oil (unrefined, cold pressed)
- Olivado: Avocado Oil (extra virgin, cold pressed)
- Rejuvenative Foods organic cold pressed oils

Naked Necessities

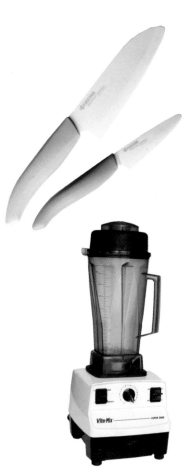

Knives

Good knives are key to happiness in the kitchen and equally important for preserving the integrity of foods. They will not only make your preparation time easier, but will cause less damage to the flesh of plant foods and will help stabilize the nutritional value for longer periods. Try Kyocera ceramic knives–they are the new craze, and are fairly inexpensive and light. I also like Global® Knives, but any fine, sharp knife that suits your grip will do.

Blender

A quality, high-speed blender is key to many Get Naked recipes. It may seem like a hefty investment at first, but when you realize the upside, you won't believe you've ever lived without it. I prefer the Vita-Mix® blender. It will actually break down the food to such a degree that your digestive system will feel relieved. The Vita-Mix® is such a powerful blender it does all the work for you, allowing vital nutrients to absorb quickly and efficiently. Another great feature of the Vita-Mix® is the warmth it brings to foods, from the friction when you leave it running. It is great for raw soups if you like them slightly heated.

Food Processor

A food processor is a staple to all kitchens. If you don't own one already, go get one. It cuts preparation time down to a minimum, and is an exceptional tool with all its gadgets for shredding, slicing, etc. I use it most often with the s-blade to mix things like veggie burgers, piecrusts, and brownies. My brand of choice is a Cuisinart®, 16-cup size. There are times when I need smaller portions, but for someone with a family of five, this size tends to suit me well.

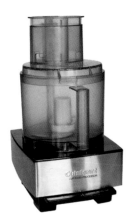

Dehydrator

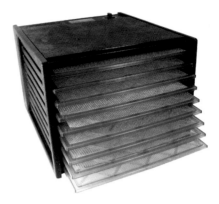

Dehydrators are an excellent way of serving your raw food warm but not cooked. It dehydrates on varied temperatures and can be used for many food items. Dehydrated nuts, vegetables, and fruits make a great snack. I prepare my raw cookies on a low temperature in the dehydrator. The brand I love is the Excalibur® Dehydrator because of its organized ParaFlexx® sheets that aid in preparing things in style. It's compact, fairly inexpensive, and easy to maintain. The dehydrator is also great for leftover fruits, vegetables, and herbs. It's so easy: just slice and dehydrate. Another innovative idea is creating fruit leathers by simply pouring your leftover smoothie onto a ParaFlexx® sheet and dehydrating. For a meal on the go, try the same with soups.

Coffee-spice/nut grinder

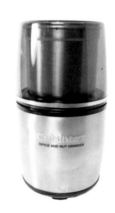

I love my Cuisinart spice and nut grinder. Since I discovered this little gem, I use it for everything. It comes with a large cup holder for bigger batches of grinding. I use it for flax seeds, sunflower seeds, grinding spices into a powder, or making raw pine nut parmesan.

Cold Coffee Press

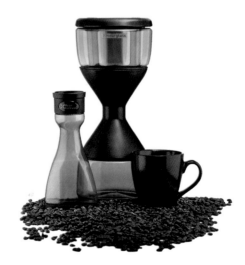

Coffee is notoriously the hardest thing to avoid when getting Naked (I must admit I love the taste of coffee). The great thing about the Hourglass® Coffee System is that it cold brews your favorite coffee into such a beautifully smooth, low acid coffee that you won't ever have to give it up. I'm really impressed with this device—it's very easy to use and makes enough coffee concentrate to last me a few days.

Rice Cooker

This is a brilliant invention, especially if you have one with a warming cycle. The automatic setting makes it convenient for cooking grains and legumes without having to hang around the house. If you have one with a timer, even better. Zojirushi® is always a good brand to use. You can prepare your morning cereal the night before and have it warm and ready for breakfast. I don't eat very much cooked food, but a rice cooker sure comes in handy when I am preparing for guests.

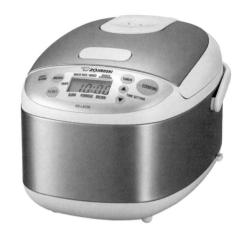

Salad Spinner

I love my salad spinner! Even though it's not a necessity, it certainly makes life easy for a quick wash and dry of your produce. Vegetables and herbs will crisp and perk up when washed, dried, and refrigerated for a few hours—great for a crunchy salad!

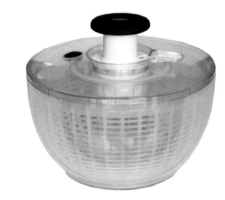

Mandoline

This tool has various settings that create a perfect shape every time. It is great for slicing beets, turnips, carrots and sweet potatoes. I use it to thinly slice my vegetables for raw raviolis.

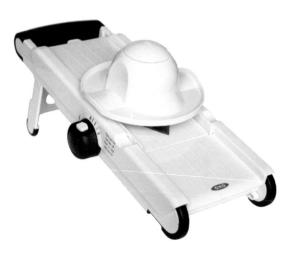

Spiralizer (or Saladacco)

This is a handheld gadget, great for making unique, stylish vegetable dishes, including shapely and delicious raw pastas. One setting makes paper-thin slices while the other produces clouds of spaghetti-like strands. I prepare yellow squash, zucchini, and beets for an angel hair pasta. You will be surprised at how creative you can get with this fun vegetable slicer!

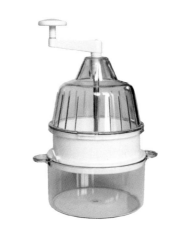

Mesh Strainers

I have many mesh strainers in different sizes. I use them to air-dry my fresh produce and also to sprout most of my seeds and legumes. For easy sprouting, just soak, rinse, and run under water through mesh strainer until sprouting tails form. It's a super easy way to instant nutrition and very ALIVE food.

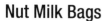

Nut Milk Bags

If you like a creamy delicious milk-like drink, you'll want to have a couple nut milk bags on hand. This reusable necessity is made with a fine mesh and meant for straining your nut milks to make them very smooth. I make many different flavors of nut milks and then store them in mason jars in my refrigerator, so my nut milk bags are in constant use. The great thing about nut milks is that when mixed with frozen bananas in the blender, they make a thick delicious nut milk shake that is full of nutrition.

"If you can organize your kitchen, you can organize your life."
~ Louis Parrisch

Sprouter

This is a bonus if you're serious about your health and understand that sprouts are a beneficial, high-energy food. It may not be easy to find fresh sprouts locally or at your convenience, but it is very easy to grow them in your kitchen. I use Freshlife® Automatic Sprouter from Tribest® in my kitchen.

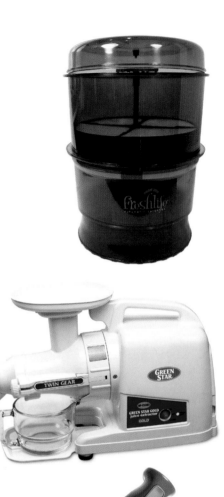

Juicer

Personally, I need to have a quart of green juice every day. I will juice anything and everything for maximum flavor and nutrition. It nourishes me and oxygenates my blood; I crave it and can't wait to drink it. My favorite juicer is a Green Star®, but there are certainly other popular ones on the market that will do the job. I'm not picky about this because I think it's better to have any ol' juicer than none at all.

Hand/Immersion Blender

One of my favorite pieces of equipment for making pureed soups and mineral broths, I also use it for whipping nut milks into a froth for a green tea latte. Inexpensive and handy, I highly suggest having one around the kitchen for ease and versatility.

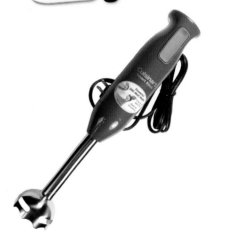

Diana's Basic Ingredients to Health, Beauty, and Longevity

Eat an 80% Raw-Vegan Diet because...

- The body is bio-electric; "live" (uncooked, unprocessed) food regenerates the electrical energy
- Raw plant proteins are readily available and easily absorbed in the cells
- Raw plant foods are laden with life force energy and enzymatic activity
- Cooking food destroys 50% of all proteins and 100% of all enzymes
- Enzymes are vital controllers, transforming food into essential substances for the body
- At a certain age, bodies no longer produce enzymes and therefore must replenish enzymes through the consumption of live food
- The link between aging and the depletion of enzymes has proven that live foods have a youth-producing effect
- Eating a vegan diet will lower your carbon footprint by 80%—even more if eating raw

Eat a Low Glycemic Diet and Avoid Artificial Sweeteners because...

- Stabilized blood sugar levels reduce the risk of heart disease and diabetes
- Sugar raises the insulin level and suppresses the immune system, increasing vulnerability to disease
- Cancer cells thrive on glucose
- Sugar ages the skin by changing the structure of collagen and causing cross-linking, a.k.a. wrinkles
- Artificial sweeteners enter the body as a poison and research has shown them to cause cancer
- Artificial sweeteners engorge the lymphatic system, storing the chemical poisons to protect vital organs from harm

Eat a Diet High in Minerals because...

- Minerals are essential to the survival of the human body, even more important than enzymes
- The primary role of minerals is to aid detoxification; many people are so low in minerals they cannot detoxify

- Humans take in their minerals from plants, plants extract their minerals from the mineral-rich soil
- Mineral deficiency often results in premature aging, fatigue, illness, and disease

Eat Foods High in Water because…

- Water is life force energy
- High-water foods are easier to digest and help flush wastes and toxins while transporting nutrients and oxygen
- Our bodies are made up of 65-75% water, and when depleted may lose energy
- Water aids digestion, but water with meals dilutes the digestive enzymes in saliva

Do Not Overeat because…

- Overeating slows the metabolism and causes premature aging
- KiSS (Keep it Simple Sweetie)—too much food confuses and overworks the digestive system
- With a nutrient-dense live food diet, fewer calories need to be consumed for nutritional fulfillment

Eat Only When Hungry because…

- If you listen to your body, it will tell you exactly what it needs
- Eating when tired, anxious, or angry changes the energy of the food, causing bodily stress
- Eating when emotionally upset causes cravings for addictive comfort/junk foods
- Comfort/junk foods create acidity in the body

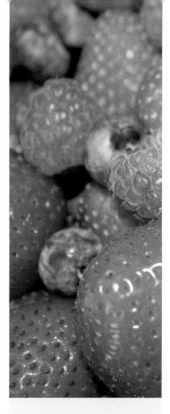

Live Naturally, Eat Naturally

Eat to feel good.

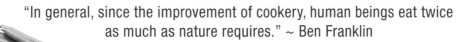

"In general, since the improvement of cookery, human beings eat twice as much as nature requires." ~ Ben Franklin

RECIPES

The Cleansing Day

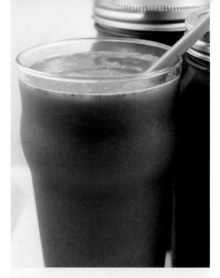

A cleansing day is much like a fasting day, except that while you are giving your body a break, you are also nourishing it with an enormous amount of minerals. Green juice cleanses are particularly powerful because they enhance the body's ability to metabolize old waste and push it through the system. It is good to do a green juice cleanse/fast once a week to keep the liver functioning properly—flushing toxins through the body. The way to do a cleanse is to make a big batch of green juice and drink it all day long, whenever you are hungry, thirsty, or just feeling like it. Water and herbal teas may also be consumed along with a handful of soaked almonds (soak for 12 hours); however, it is important to note that anything eaten, including almonds, will slow down the cleansing process. If you can drink only green juice for one day, you will feel the amazing benefits the next morning and then all week long.

I like to make Monday my cleansing day. It is the start of a new week, and if I stray from my healthy ways, it is likely to happen on a weekend. Even if I am not fasting, I like to have a quart of green juice every day around mid-morning. I make a batch of my Favorite Green Juice 3 times a week. Sometimes I have to make it every day, as my family has become quite addicted to its nutritional benefits! It can be an acquired taste for some, but it will soon become a craving that your body will yearn for.

Diana's Favorite Green Juice Cleanse

3 cucumbers

2 bunches celery

1 bunch parsley

1 bunch rainbow chard

3 green apples

3 lemons

2 fennel bulbs

Do not remove any parts of any vegetable or fruit. Push all ingredients through a juicer. This fresh juice will last 2 days in the refrigerator.

Makes 4 quarts

Breaking the Fast

The word "breakfast" is a combination of two words, "break" and "fast," which literally means to break your nighttime fast. The reason for breaking your fast gently is that there may still be undigested food left in your belly from the night before. It's helpful to clear that out before taxing your body with more food. A great way to break the morning fast and help eliminate anything left over in the digestive track is by drinking a large glass of water with freshly squeezed lemon juice in it before you move about your day.

I like to start my day with a smoothie for breakfast, but I realize that many people like to start their day with something hearty. We all have our favorite times to eat, and some habits are hard to break. Here are a variety of familiar and healthful choices for breakfast that can be used as guidelines to explore the range of tastes that appeal to you. Eventually, you'll find that it's nice to ease into your day with a light meal and save your larger meal for lunch.

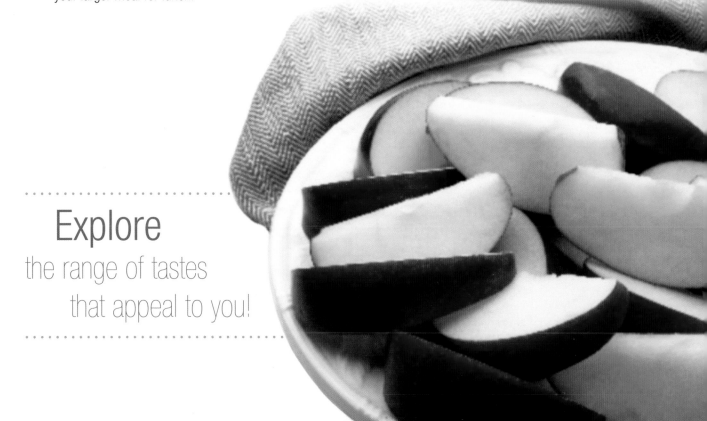

Explore
the range of tastes
that appeal to you!

Fresh Apple Muesli with Maple-Pecan Cream

Makes 1-2 servings • Prep time: 15 minutes

Fruit is one of the best things you can eat to start your morning. It moves quickly through the digestive tract and cleans out any stagnant waste. This cereal is a treat that provides the crunch and sweetness of a morning cereal, with a nice energetic boost.

Ingredients

1 apple, cored and diced

¼ cup whole raw almonds

1 tablespoon raisins

¼ teaspoon cinnamon

1 pinch of sea salt

Maple-Pecan Cream

½ cup pecans or pecan butter

½ cup water

2 tablespoons maple syrup

Blend all ingredients in high-speed blender until smooth and creamy. Extra cream will keep in refrigerator for up to 5 days, and may also be used as a dip or dessert option.

Directions

Fit processor with s-blade and mix all ingredients in processor bowl together. Pulse 12-15 times until coarsely chopped or desired consistency is obtained. For a crunchier cereal, pulse less; for a smoother texture, process longer. Transfer cereal to serving bowl and top with Maple-Pecan Cream.

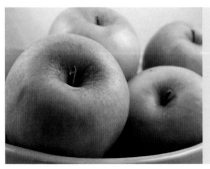

 FUN FACT: The more tart an apple, the higher it is in vitamin C.

 NUTRITIONAL BENEFIT: Apples are an excellent source of fiber.

 HOW TO SELECT: Choose apples in season that are firm and free of bruises and blemishes.

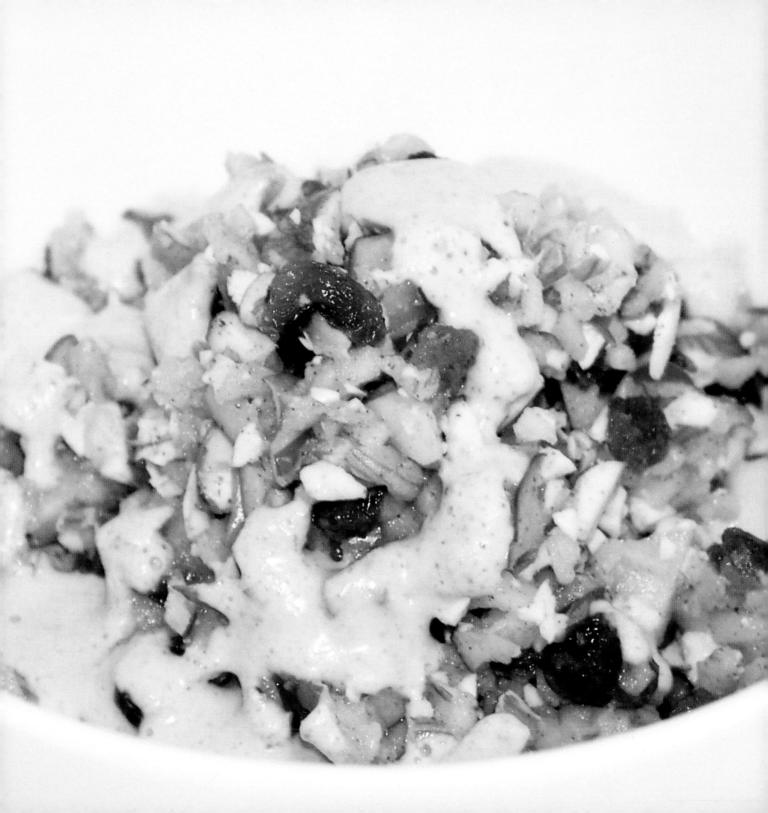

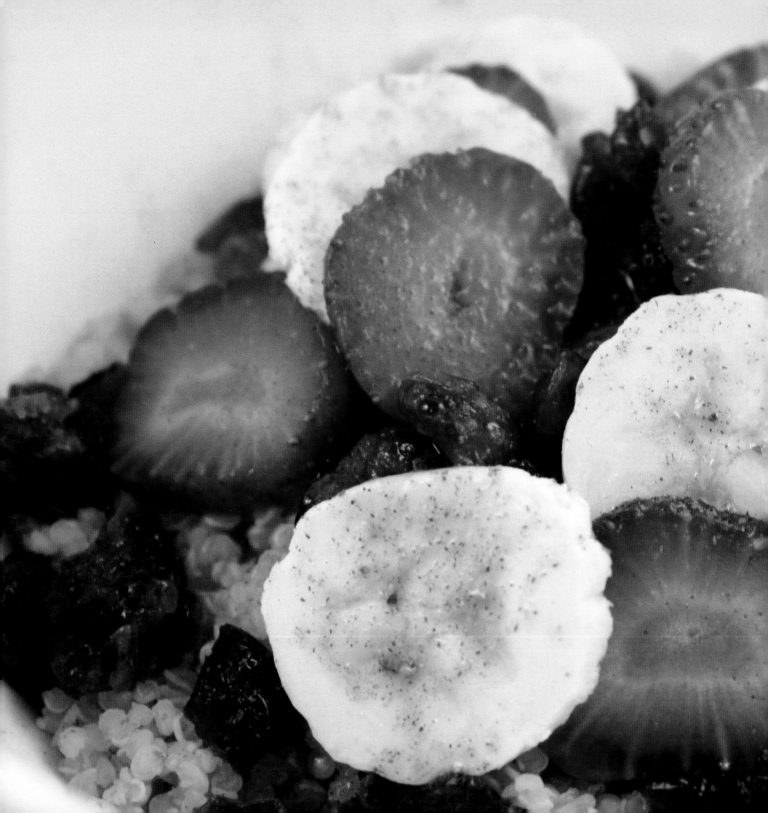

Hot Quinoa-Cranberry Cereal
with Bananas and Strawberries

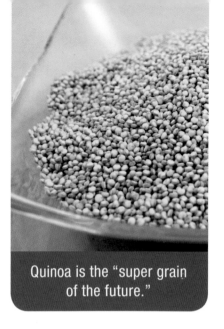

Quinoa is the "super grain of the future."

Makes 1-2 servings • Prep time: 20 minutes

A cozy, warm bowl of hot cereal is always a nice idea. This cereal is packed full of protein and delicious nutrients, and is especially good with almond milk served on the side or poured over the top.

Ingredients

1 cup quinoa

2 cups water

2 tablespoons cranberries, dried

¼ teaspoon cinnamon

1/8 teaspoon sea salt

1 banana, sliced

2-3 strawberries, sliced

agave nectar for drizzle

Directions

Place quinoa and water in a 2-quart saucepan and bring to boil. Then reduce heat to simmer; cover and let cook until all water is absorbed (10-15 minutes). When done, the grain appears translucent and the germ ring will be visible. Extra quinoa may be stored in the refrigerator in an airtight container for up to 5 days. Use for other recipes.

Scoop one cup of hot, cooked quinoa into serving bowl. Serve with cranberries, bananas, and strawberries, then drizzle with agave nectar and sprinkle with cinnamon.

Optional: Use a rice cooker and prepare the night before. The rice cooker will hold at a warming cycle until morning.

Basic Almond Milk

Makes 3-4 servings • Prep time: 5 minutes

You'll want this one in your fridge at all times; it's perfect to drink as milk or as a base for your smoothies. Prepare a fresh batch every 3-4 days.

Ingredients

1 cup whole raw almonds, soaked in water 12 hours

4 cups purified water

Directions

Drain and rinse almonds. Place in high-speed blender with water and blend until completely broken down and a milky color appears. Place nut milk bag into large pitcher or bowl. Pour nut milk mixture into bag. Close bag and gently squeeze with hands until all liquid is extracted. The remaining pulp may be discarded or frozen in an airtight container.

....

Whole almonds with skins provide heart-healthy benefits.

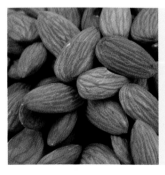

 FUN FACT: The ancient Romans showered newlyweds with almonds as a fertility charm.

 NUTRITIONAL BENEFIT: The highest amount of protein of all nuts, supporting healthy mind and bones.

 HOW TO SELECT: Look for almonds that are uniform in color and smell sweet.

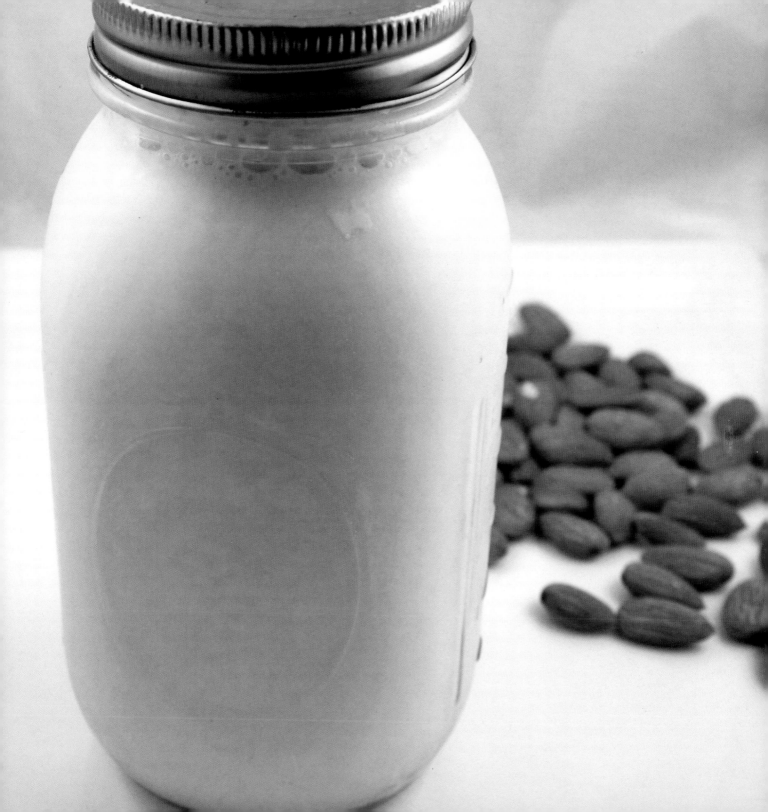

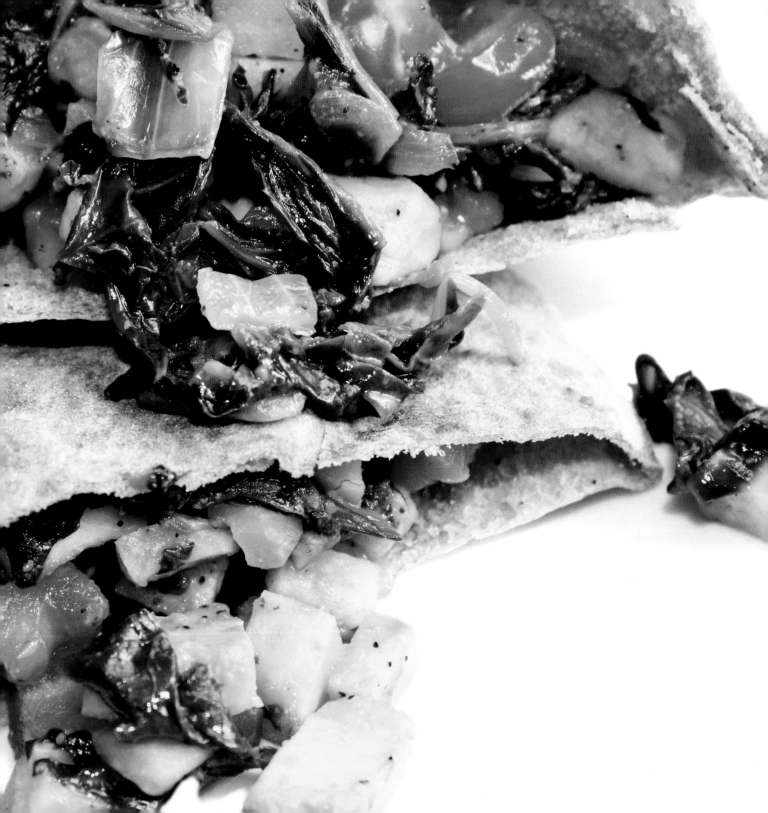

Veggie Hash Pockets

Makes 1-2 servings   •   Prep time: 15 minutes

This is a great breakfast option for hearty breakfast eaters. Kohlrabi and celery root each have thick skin that can be eaten, but it's better to peel or cut off the skin before dicing.

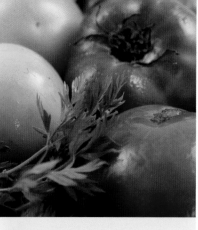

Ingredients

- 1-2 sprouted grain pita pockets
- ½ cup onion, diced (approx. ½ onion)
- ½ cup kohlrabi, fennel bulb, or celery root, diced (approx. ½ bulb or root)
- 2 cups spinach, shredded
- 1 medium tomato, diced
- ½ avocado, diced
- 1 tablespoon ghee
- sea salt
- black pepper

FUN FACT: Botanically, tomatoes are actually berries.

NUTRITIONAL BENEFIT: Tomatoes are high in lycopene, which flush free radicals.

HOW TO SELECT: Fragrance is a better indicator of a good tomato than color.

Directions

Sauté onion and kohlrabi (or fennel or celery root) in ghee until tender. Add spinach and briefly sauté until wilted. Add tomato and avocado until heated, and then season with salt and pepper to taste. Cut pita pocket in half, toast lightly, then fill each half with Veggie Hash.

Banana Buckwheat Pancakes
with Cinnamon Agave Drizzle

Makes 8 pancakes • Prep time: 30 minutes

These are so decadent, you may want to save this recipe for your Sunday morning breakfast splurge. But, no worries—they are packed full of protein and good nutrients.

Ingredients

1 cup cooked quinoa

½ cup buckwheat flour

1 ripe banana

1 cup almond milk

2 teaspoons raw honey

1 teaspoon baking soda

1 teaspoon baking powder

extra virgin coconut oil for frying

Agave Drizzle

Ingredients

1 tablespoon agave

½ teaspoon cinnamon

To prepare quinoa:

Place 1 cup quinoa and 2 cups water in 2-quart saucepan; bring to boil. Reduce heat to simmer then cover and let cook until all water is absorbed (10-15 minutes). When done, the grain appears translucent and the germ ring will be visible. Quinoa may be prepared the night before or used from leftovers.

To prepare pancakes:

Fit processor with s-blade and mix quinoa, buckwheat, banana, almond milk, honey, baking soda, and baking powder together until batter is smooth. Melt 1-2 teaspoons coconut oil in nonstick pan over medium-high heat. Pour approximately 1/3 cup of batter per pancake into 4-inch rounds. Cook until edges are firm (about 2 minutes). Flip pancake and cook for 1 additional minute. To serve, place on a plate and drizzle with Agave Drizzle. Garnish with fresh banana slices.

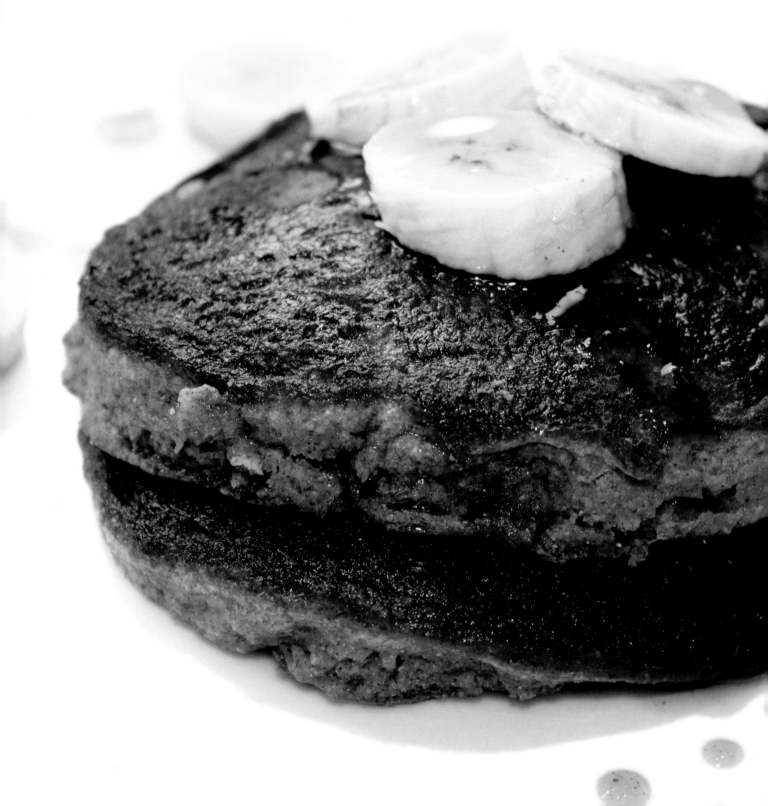

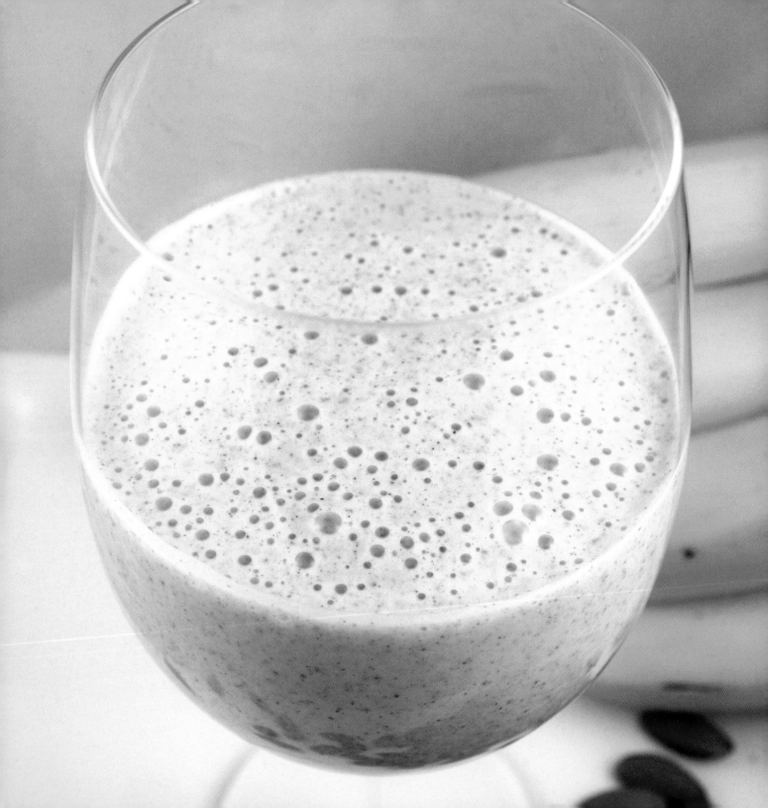

Easy Almond Date Milkshake

Makes 1 serving • Prep time: 2 minutes

No almond milk on hand? This perfect morning shake is quick and easy. Feel free to add green powders, superfoods, honey, and fresh fruits for an energy boost and flavor variety.

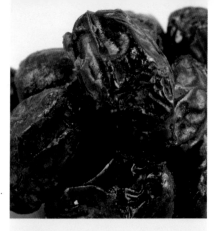

Ingredients

2 tablespoons raw almond butter

2 Medjool dates, pitted

1½ cups cold water

1 frozen banana

Directions

Blend all ingredients in high-speed blender for 30-40 seconds until creamy.

FUN FACT: Dates are the sweetest fruit.

NUTRITIONAL BENEFIT: Dates contain more potassium than bananas, and provide instant energy.

HOW TO SELECT: Look for moist, plump dates.

Frozen bananas are great for thickening smoothies.

Popeye's Passion

Makes 1 serving • Prep time: less than 5 minutes

This is an all-time favorite, power-packed green smoothie.

Ingredients

2 cups fresh pressed apple juice

2 cups fresh organic spinach

1 frozen banana

Directions

Blend all ingredients in high-speed blender for 30-40 seconds until creamy. Enjoy immediately.

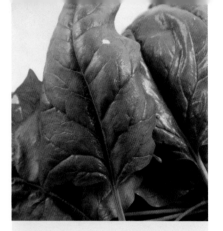

FUN FACT: Spinach belongs to the goosefoot family along with beets and chard.

NUTRITIONAL BENEFIT: Spinach contains more protein than any other vegetable.

HOW TO SELECT: Choose spinach with tender, green leaves.

A muscle-building plant protein, spinach also has high levels of calcium, iron, vitamins A, C, and E as well as antioxidants.

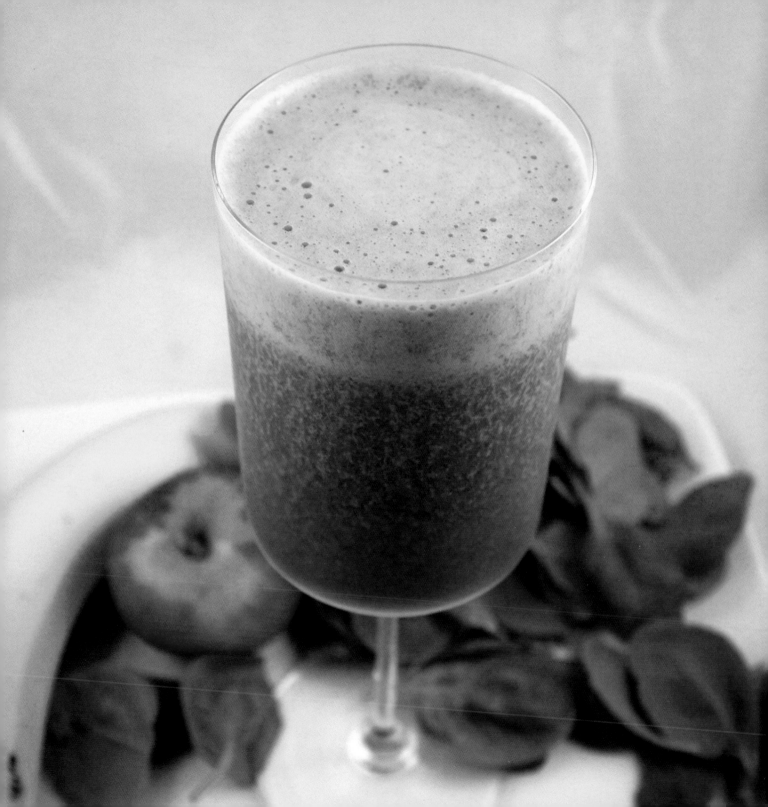

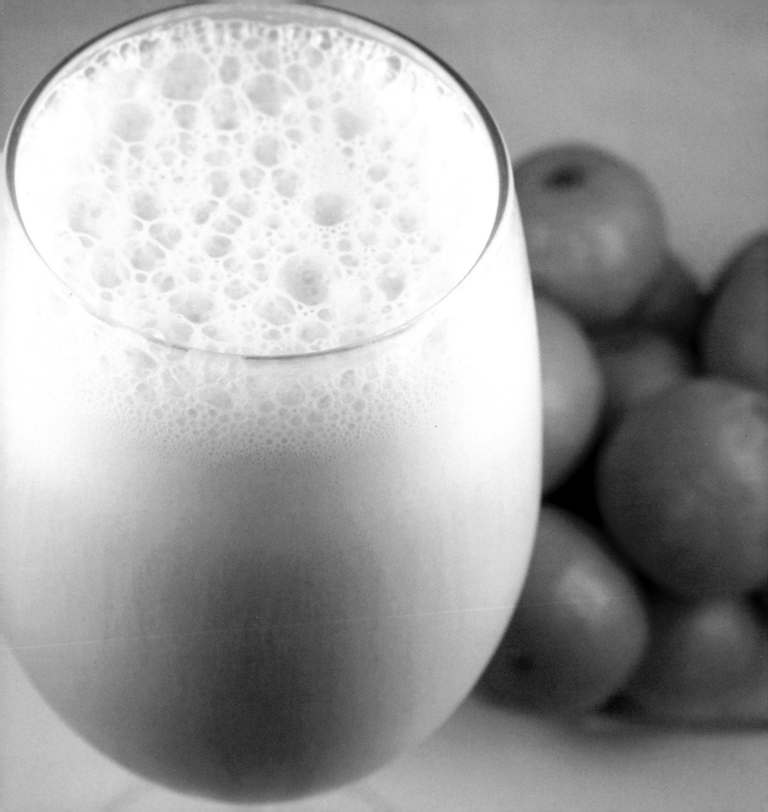

Julius Kefir Smoothie

Makes 1 serving • Prep time: 2-5 minutes

A long time favorite, kefir is the only dairy product I allow in my regime. Try using only freshly squeezed orange juice for freshness, flavor, and ultimate nutrition.

Ingredients

1 cup orange juice, freshly squeezed

1 cup kefir, vanilla flavor

1 frozen banana

Directions

Blend all ingredients in high-speed blender for 30-40 seconds until creamy.

Kefir contains lots of good bacteria for your intestines.

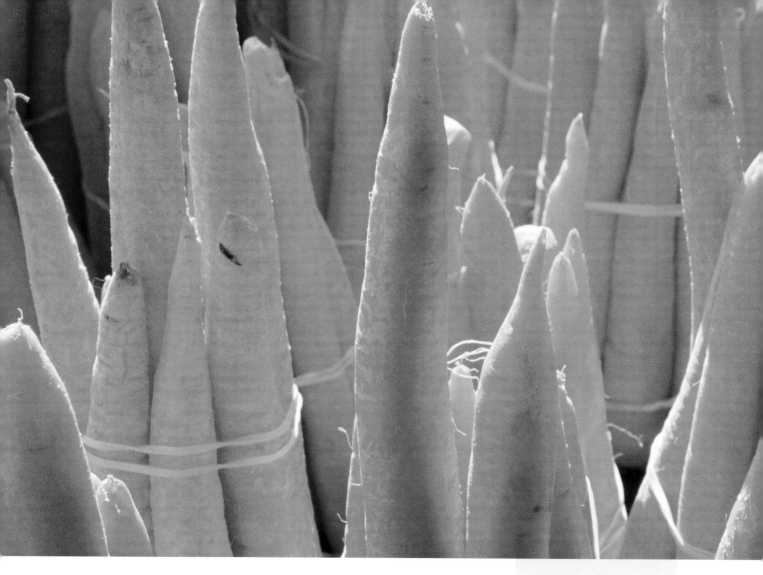

Foods That Nourish the Tummy

- Artichokes
- Avocados
- Barley
- Brown Rice
- Carrots
- Millet Sprouts
- Parsnips
- Squash
- Sweet Potatoes
- Turnips
- Yams

Teas/Herbs

- Fennel
- Peppermint
- Licorice

Lite Energy Meals

According to our biorhythms, it's best to eat your largest meal at lunchtime. Getting Naked means never being weighed down by overeating, so a large meal is something you will learn to balance out over time. These lunch recipes provide some delicious, easy-to-make choices that will satiate your mid-day hunger. Many of the foods can be prepared ahead and packaged for work, or assembled when it's time to eat. Take advantage of the many live food options for lunchtime, as you want the vital energy of plant food to keep you energized throughout the day.

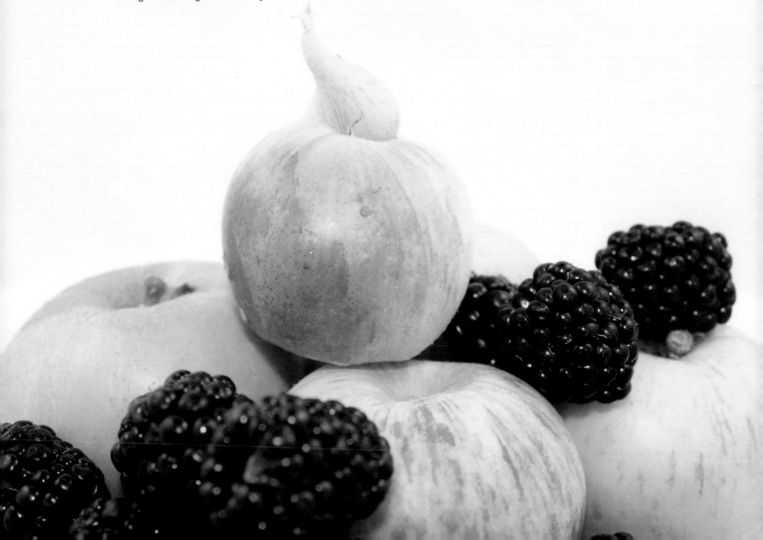

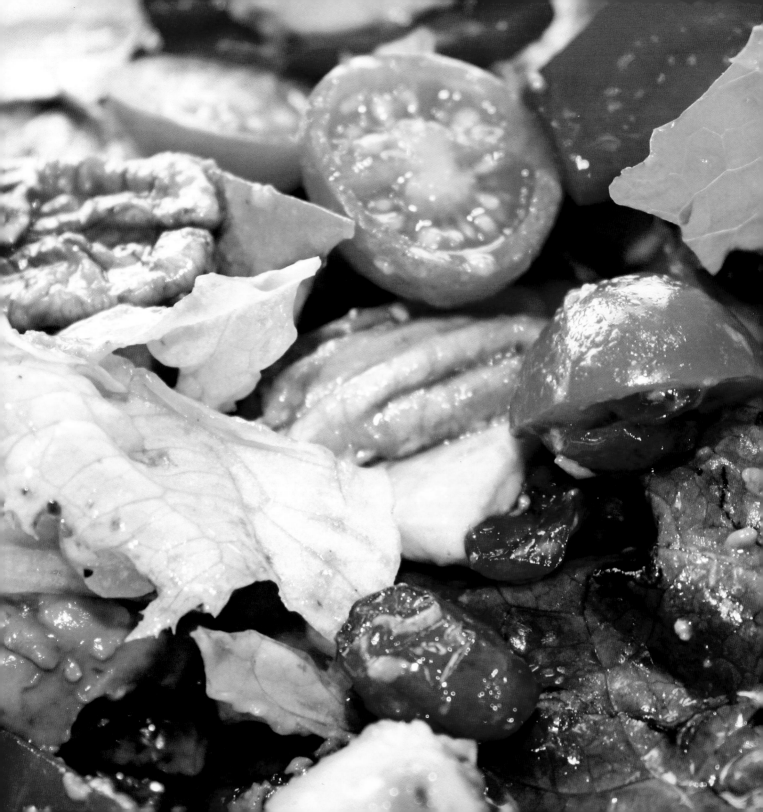

The Really Big Salad

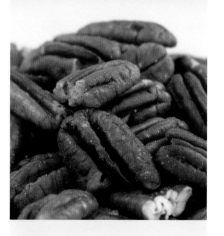

Makes 1 serving • Prep time: 10 minutes

This is a naked version of a salad I used to eat in a café in Berkeley, California. Make it really big and enjoy it often. Add fresh figs or chopped fresh herbs for a boost of minerals and variety.

Ingredients

½ head of romaine or red leaf lettuce, shredded

1 medium beet, thinly sliced or grated

½ avocado, diced

10 cherry tomatoes, halved

2 tablespoons cranberries, dried

2 tablespoons raw pecan halves

1 tablespoon flaxseed oil or Udo's Choice™ Oil Blend

1 tablespoon fig balsamic vinegar

sea salt

black pepper

FUN FACT: The U.S. produces 80% of the world's pecans.

NUTRITIONAL BENEFIT: Pecans are said to increase sexual desire due to their zinc content.

HOW TO SELECT: Select plump pecans that are uniform in size and color.

Directions

Place shredded lettuce, beets, avocado and tomatoes in a large salad bowl. Sprinkle with cranberries and pecans. Drizzle with oil and vinegar, and add salt and pepper to taste.

Lettuce aids digestion and promotes liver health.

Butternut Squash Soup

Makes 4-6 servings • Prep time: 30 minutes

This simple and delicious soup is a staple in my home, a favorite amongst my friends, and a recipe I give out often. It's a smooth, warm and satisfying meal that can be made in advance. For a heartier version, serve with flax crackers.

Ingredients

4 cups butternut squash, peeled and diced (approx. 1 medium squash)

1 large yellow onion, diced

2 tablespoons ghee

1 quart Pacific Foods organic vegetable broth

1½ teaspoons sea salt

1 pinch of saffron threads or powder (optional)

Flaxseed oil or Udo's Choice™ Oil Blend for drizzle

Directions

In 4-quart saucepan, sauté onion and butternut squash in ghee until vegetables sweat, but do not brown. Add vegetable broth, saffron, and sea salt. Cook on medium/low heat until vegetables are tender and soft, about 15 minutes. Turn off heat and cool slightly. Place immersion blender directly in pot and blend until pureed, or to desired consistency.

If you do not have an immersion blender, cool and transfer mixture to standard blender and puree for 20-30 seconds. Return mixture to saucepan and bring back to desired heat. To serve, ladle into bowls and drizzle with flaxseed oil or Udo's Choice™ Oil Blend.

....

Flaxseed oil eases weight loss and increases metabolism

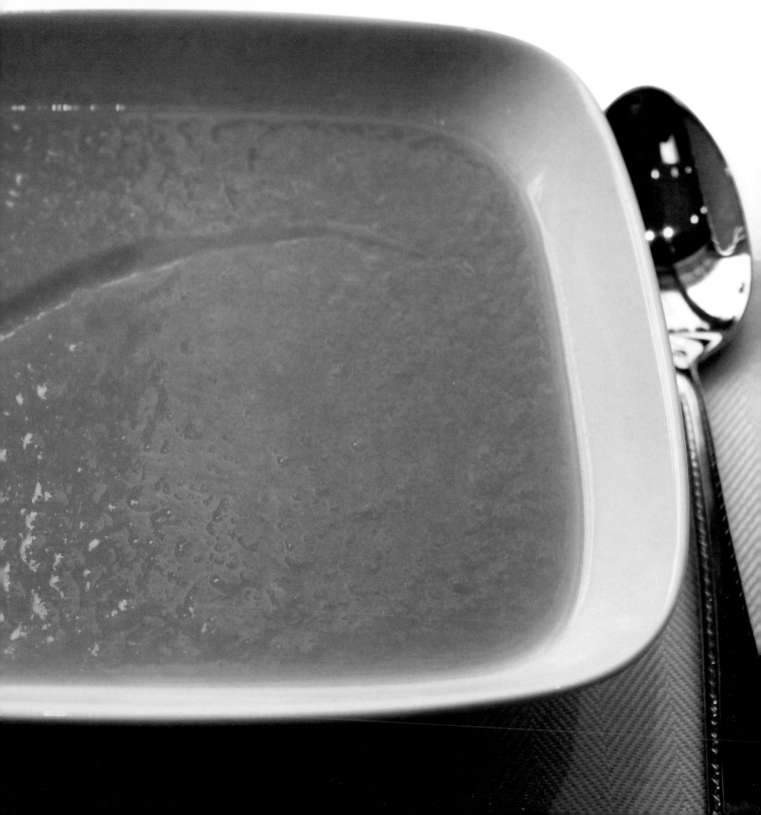

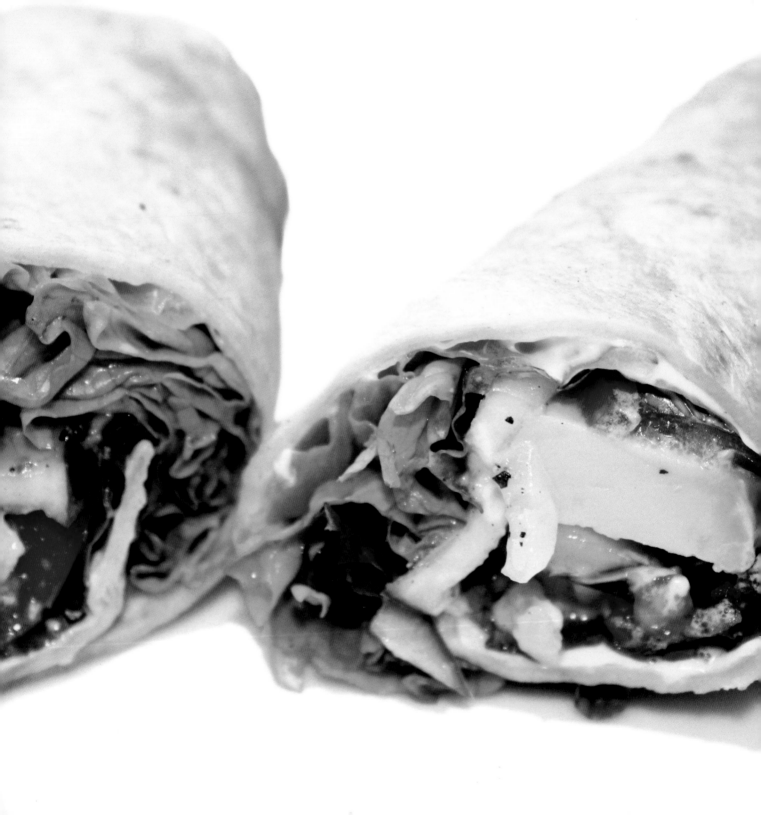

ALT Wrap
with Fresh Sweet Pickles

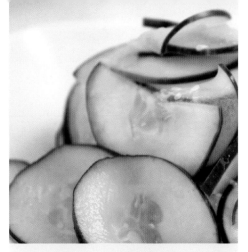

Makes 1 serving • Prep time: 5 minutes

Avocado, Lettuce and Tomato Wraps—one bite, and you'll be hooked! Easy and satisfying, this is a great meal to take on the go. You will want to prepare the pickles in advance.

Ingredients

1 spelt or sprouted grain tortilla

½ avocado, sliced

2 leaves of hearts of romaine or red leaf lettuce

5 cherry tomatoes, halved

Vegenaise

sea salt

black pepper

To prepare wrap:

Assemble wrap by laying tortilla flat while placing vegetables, pickles, and seasoning on top. Roll tortilla, manipulating vegetables tightly into the wrap. Slice in half and serve.

Sweet Pickles

Ingredients

1 cucumber, sliced

2 tablespoons agave nectar

1 tablespoon apple cider vinegar

1 tablespoon Ume plum vinegar

To prepare pickles:

Place sliced cucumbers in an airtight container. Add vinegars and agave and cover with lid. Shake to incorporate flavors, then let marinate overnight in refrigerator.

Vegenaise is an egg-free mayonnaise made with good oils.
It is found in the refrigerator section of your local health food store.

Open Face Hummus Sandwich

Makes 1 serving • Prep time: less than 5 minutes

You may have this sandwich two-faced, as well, but two slices of bread may be filling. This is a great meal for traveling or when you're on the go. Try rolling it in a tortilla for variation. To make this easy to grab and go, prepare the hummus and pickles in advance.

Ingredients

1-2 slices sprouted grain bread, toasted if desired

Zucchini Hummus (page 67) for raw version, or hummus of your choice

½ cucumber, sliced

½ avocado, sliced

½ tomato, sliced

sprouts or lettuce

Onion Pickles

To prepare sandwich:

Spread Zucchini Hummus on top of bread slices and layer avocado, cucumber, and tomato slices.
Add lettuce or sprouts and top with Onion Pickles.

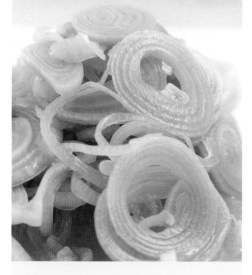

Onion Pickles

Ingredients

1 onion, thinly sliced

2 teaspoons Ume plum vinegar

2 teaspoons apple cider vinegar

Directions:

Place onions in airtight container, add vinegars and cover with lid. Shake to incorporate flavors, then let marinate overnight in refrigerator.

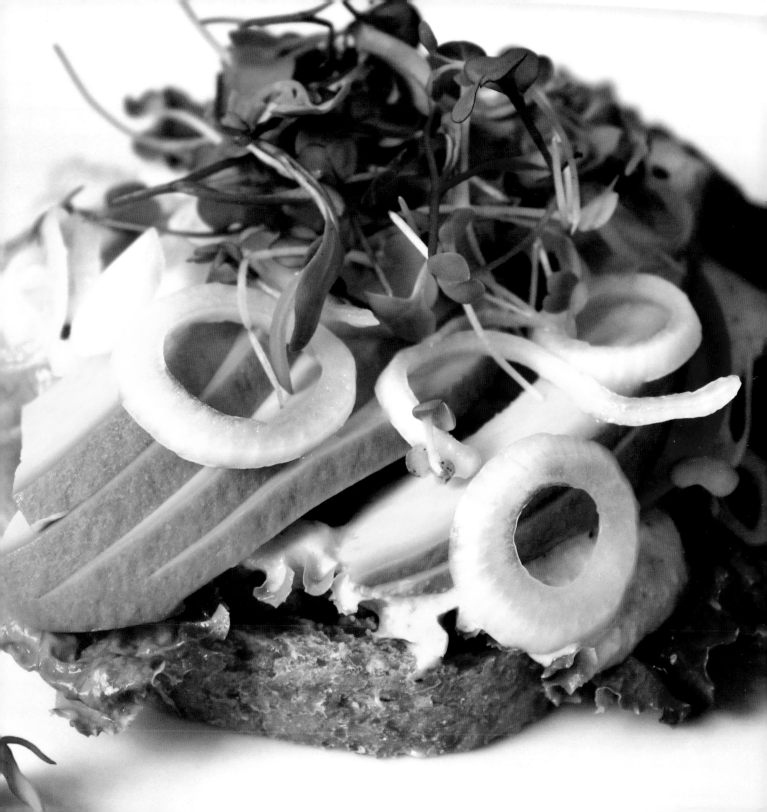

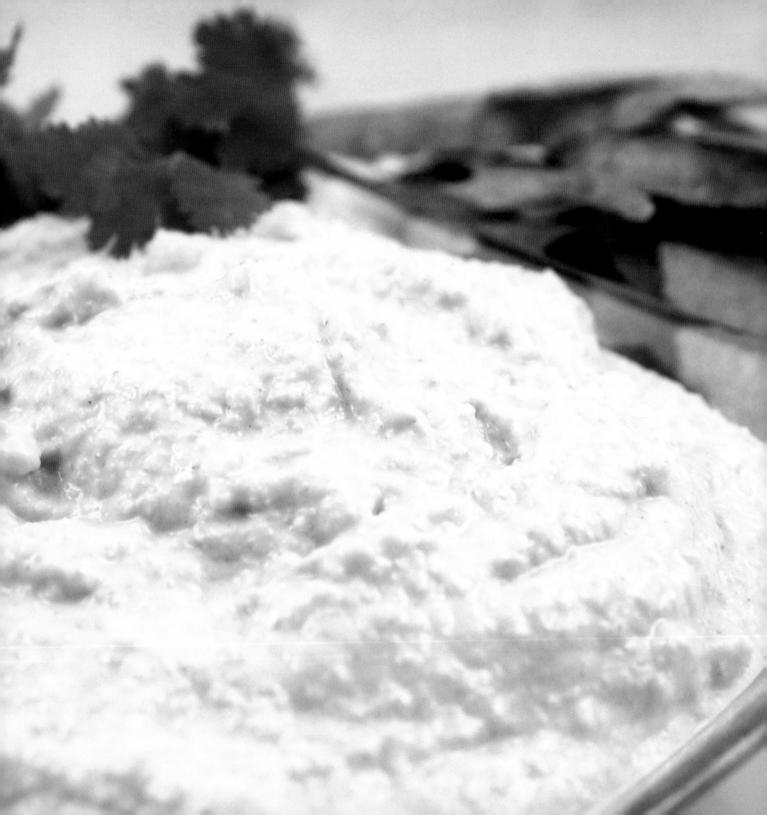

Zucchini Hummus

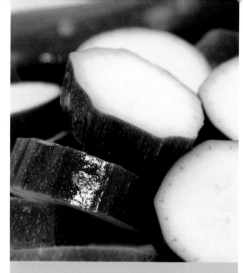

Makes 3 cups • Prep time: 5 minutes

Ingredients

2 cups zucchini, diced (approximately 2 zucchinis)

¾ cup tahini

½ cup lemon juice, freshly squeezed

¼ cup olive oil

1 clove garlic, minced

1½ teaspoons sea salt

2 teaspoons cumin powder

Definitely wash your zucchini, but don't peel—most of the nutrients are in the skin.

Directions:

In food processor fitted with s-blade, process all ingredients until smooth. Store in airtight container in refrigerator for up to 5 days.

Most prepared hummus are made with canned chickpeas, which are stripped of vitamins and acidic in nature.

My Big Fat Greek Salad

Makes 2 servings • Prep time: 10 minutes

*Zucchini hummus gives this salad a big, fat Greek twist!
It's super easy, elegant, and delicious.*

Ingredients

1 head romaine lettuce, chopped

1 cucumber, diced

1 large tomato, wedged or diced

1 red bell pepper, sliced

½ red onion, sliced thin

¼ cup raw kalamata olives, pitted and chopped

¼ cup Zucchini Hummus (page 67)

To prepare salad:
Place all salad fixings together in large salad bowl. Drizzle with
Dressing and serve with scoops of Zucchini Hummus.

Dressing

Ingredients

½ cup olive oil

¼ cup lemon juice freshly
squeezed

2 teaspoons fresh oregano
leaves, crushed (or ½
teaspoon dried oregano)

½ teaspoon sea salt

freshly ground black
pepper (to taste)

Directions:

Mix all ingredients together.
Store extra dressing in the
refrigerator for up to 5 days.

Truly raw olives are loaded with vitamin E, a great antioxidant that neutralizes free radicals in the body.

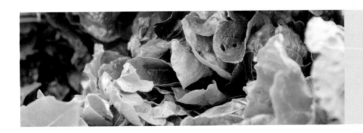

Darker green lettuce leaves means
more nutrition in your salad.

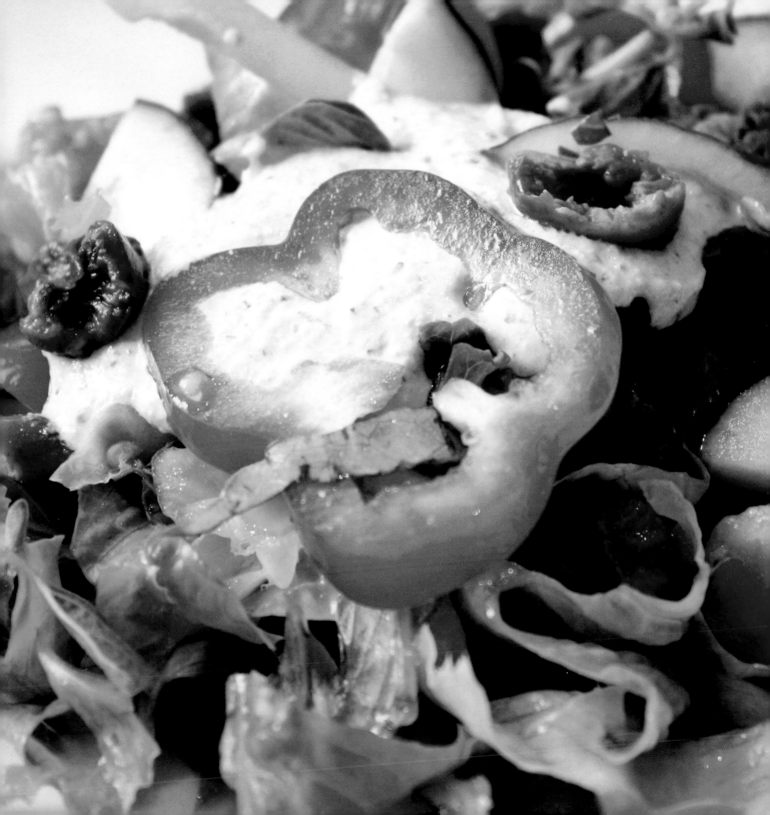

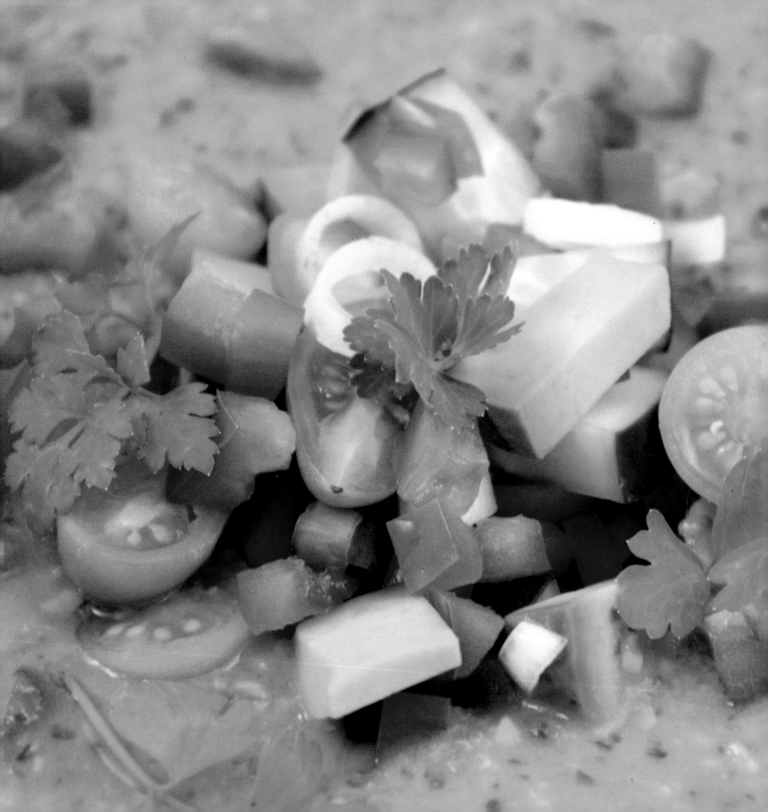

Avo Gazpacho Mexicana

Makes 2 servings • Prep time: 10 minutes

If you like cold soups, this one will rock your world! Packed with beautifying minerals, active enzymes, and phytonutrients, this soup will make your energy soar and lift you up into the later part of your day.

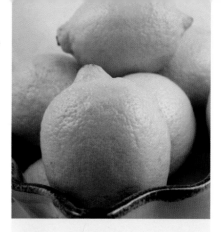

Ingredients

- 1 large avocado, diced
- ½ cucumber, diced
- ½ cup fresh cilantro leaves
- ½ cup purified water
- 1 scallion, chopped
- 10-20 cherry tomatoes, halved
- ½ red bell pepper, diced
- ½ jalapeño pepper, seeded and diced
- 1 teaspoon cumin, ground
- 1½ tablespoons lemon juice, freshly squeezed (juice of 1 lemon)
- ½ teaspoon sea salt

FUN FACT: Lemons at room temperature will yield more juice.

NUTRITIONAL BENEFIT: Lemons are high in vitamin C and fiber, and help stimulate the liver.

HOW TO SELECT: Look for lemons that are heavy for their size and have a fine-textured peel.

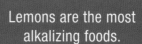

Lemons are the most alkalizing foods.

Directions

Reserve a small portion each of avocado, cucumber, cilantro, red pepper, tomato, and scallion. Mix these ingredients together and arrange in a mound in the center of two separate soup bowls. Place remaining ingredients in high-speed blender and blend on low for 15-30 seconds. Pay attention to consistency: blend more if you like it pureed, and less if you like it a bit chunky. Pour directly from blender over mounds of garnish in serving bowls. Serve with flax crackers or tortilla chips.

PB & J

Makes 1 serving • Prep time: less than 5 minutes

It may not be the classic peanut butter and jelly sandwich, but it sure hits the spot when you have a hankering for one. This is a delicious treat on any of your favorite non-glutenous breads, and is a healthy alternative to an American favorite.

Ingredients

1 slice sprouted grain bread, sprouted grain English muffin, or Manna Bread®

2 tablespoons raw almond butter or raw pecan butter

1-2 Medjool dates, pitted and chopped or mashed

Directions

Using fork, mash dates into a paste; add droplets of water to help with consistency. Assemble sandwich by spreading bread with nut butter and dates.

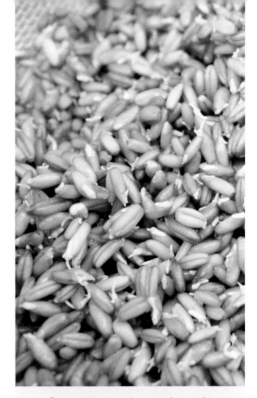

Sprouting grains and seeds before baking produces living, nutrient-rich food.

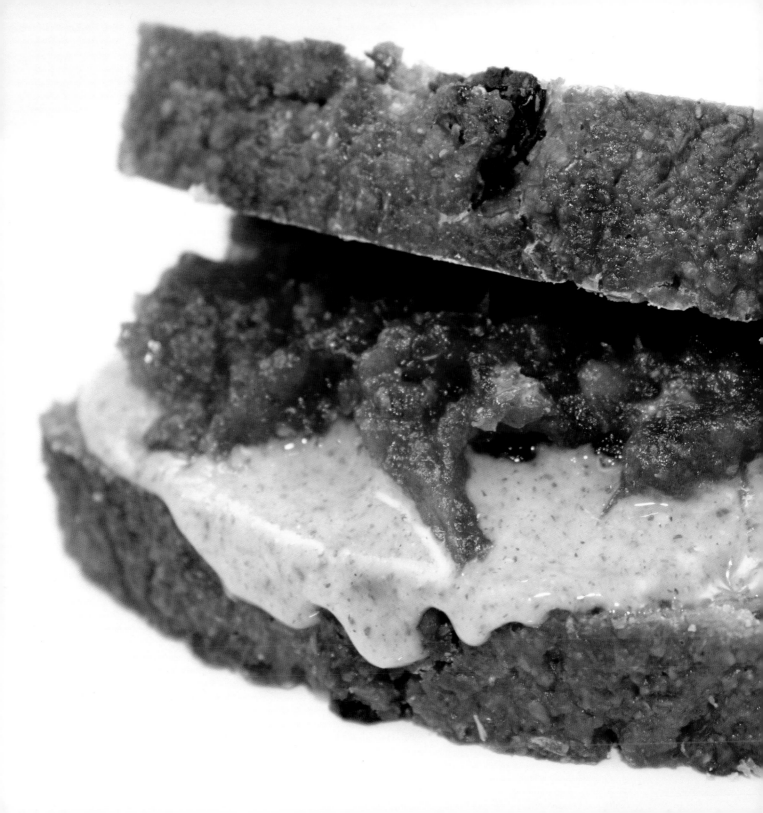

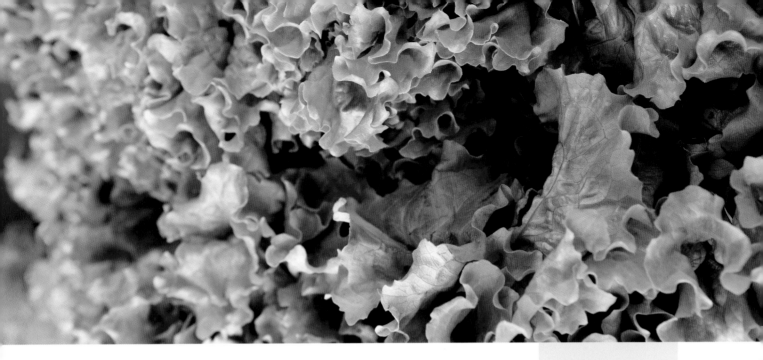

Foods That Nourish the Spleen

- Adzuki/Azuki Beans
- Yellow Squash
- Mung Beans
- Kidney Beans
- Alfalfa
- Lychees
- Barley
- Millet
- Beetroot
- Oats
- Carrots
- Parsley
- Celery
- Parsnips
- Pumpkin
- Fennel
- Sweet Potatoes
- Turnips
- Yams

High in Chlorophyll

- Leafy Greens
- Algae
- Kale
- Chard

Herbs/Spices

- Garlic
- Black Pepper
- Ginger
- Cayenne Pepper
- Ginseng
- Cinnamon
- Horseradish
- Dill Seed
- Pau d'Arco
- Astragalus

Hearty Options

I've found that most traditional dinners can feel nurturing because they are warm and cooked. I understand the need for traditional comfort, so I've included some delicious and easy *warm* (not *hot*) dishes that can help satiate the need for cooked food. But, please feel free to opt for a salad any evening, and I promise you won't regret it. It's best to keep the portions for these warm recipes to a reasonable size, as you will be sleeping on the foods (not to mention dessert) that didn't have time to work their way through your system.

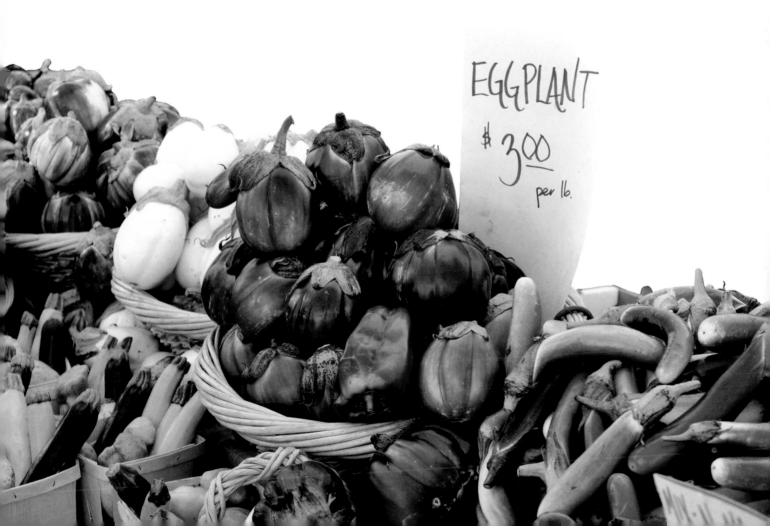

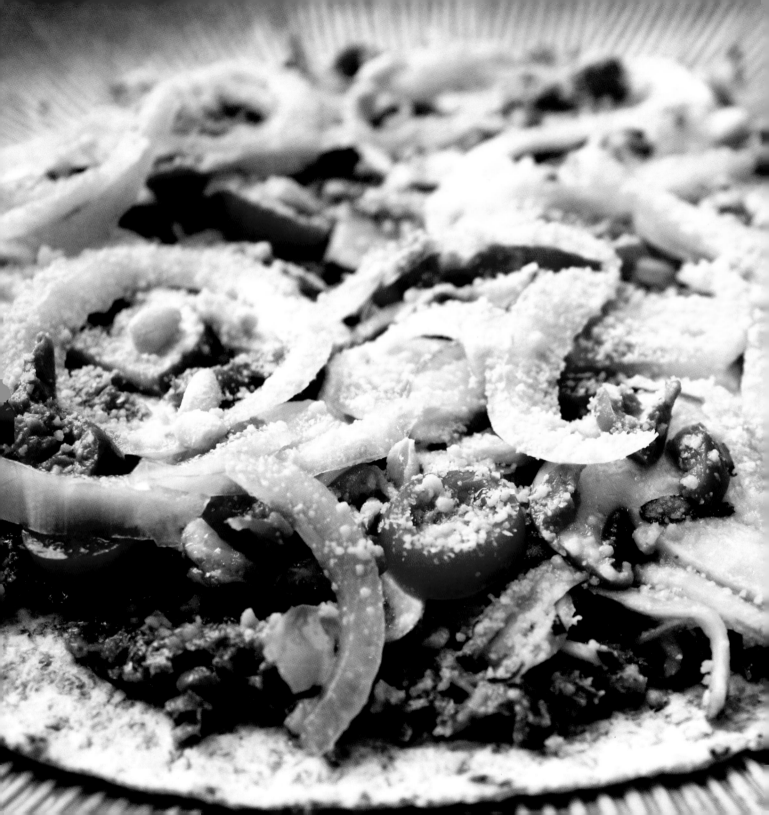

A Pesto "Cheetza"

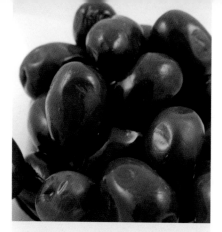

Olives are the fruit highest
in minerals and calcium.

Makes 4 pizzas • Prep time: 20-30 minutes

*This is my version of a raw pizza that's fun to make. Add any of your
favorite vegetable toppings for your own original creation. If you
have some pickled onions left over from the Open Face Hummus
Sandwich, use them in this recipe for some added tang.*

Ingredients

4 Ezekiel 4:9® Sprouted Grain Tortillas

1 recipe Pesto (page 79)

5 zucchinis, grated

8-10 mushrooms, thinly sliced

10-12 cherry tomatoes, thinly sliced

1 dozen raw kalamata olives, pitted and chopped

Bariani cold pressed olive oil

sea salt

1 recipe Pine Nut Parmesan (page 79)

To prepare "Cheetza":

Place shredded zucchini in a separate bowl. Drizzle conservatively with Bariani olive oil and sprinkle lightly with salt. Mix
and let stand to marinate.

Place sliced mushrooms in a separate bowl. Drizzle conservatively with Bariani olive oil and sprinkle lightly with salt. Mix
and let stand to marinate.

Lay tortillas on cutting board and spread approximately 1/3 cup of Pesto on each. With hands, spread approximately
1 cup of marinated zucchini evenly over the Pesto. Repeat with marinated mushrooms for the next layer, then with the
cherry tomatoes and olives. Sprinkle with Pine Nut Parmesan, then cut into four slices and enjoy.

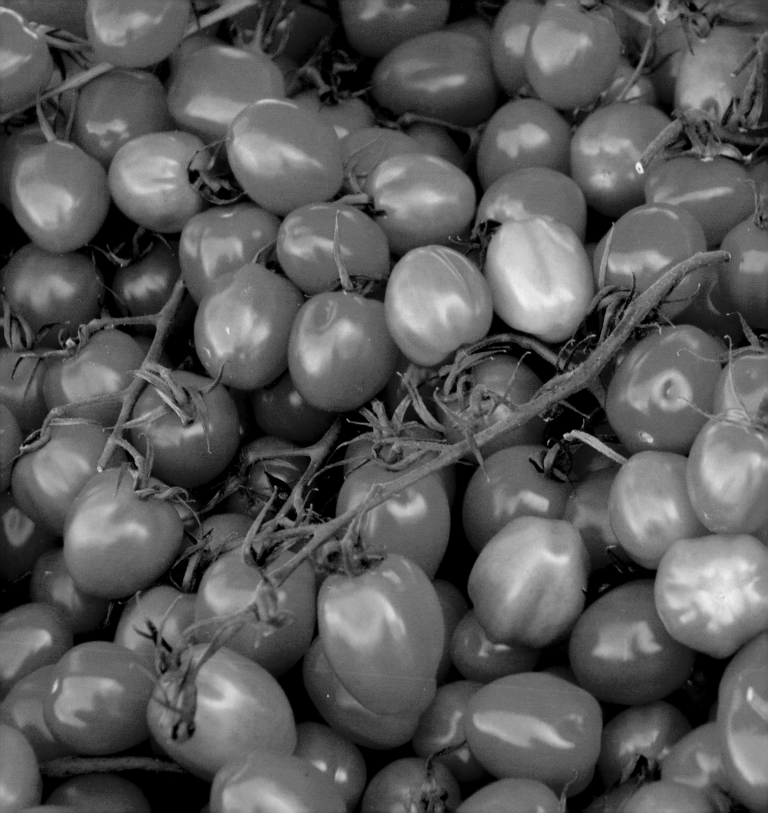

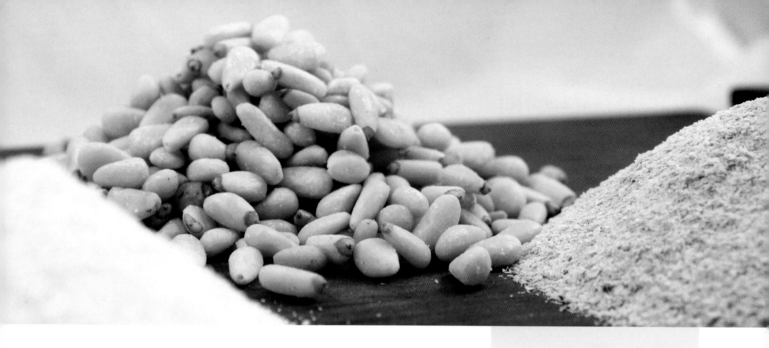

Pesto

Ingredients

2 cups fresh basil leaves, tightly packed

1 cup walnuts or pine nuts

½ cup olive oil

1 clove garlic, peeled and minced

1 tablespoon lemon juice, freshly squeezed

½ teaspoon sea salt

Directions

Place all ingredients in processor fitted with an s-blade. Pulse 10-15 times until desired consistency, scraping down sides to incorporate all the flavors. Place in bowl and set aside. Pesto can be prepared ahead of time and stored in refrigerator for up to 5 days.

Pine Nut Parmesan

Ingredients

½ cup pine nuts

¼ cup nutritional yeast

½ teaspoon sea salt

Directions

Place all ingredients in processor fitted with an s-blade. Pulse 10-12 times until flaky consistency is reached, then remove and set aside. Store excess Pine Nut Parmesan in an airtight container for later use.

Pine nuts are believed to be an appetite suppressant.

Very Teriyaki Vegetable Quinoa Bowl

Makes 1-4 servings • Prep time: 20-25 minutes

Quinoa is light, tasty, and easy to digest. It is unusually high in protein and very satisfying. Try the red Incan variation to enhance your palate. Add lots of your favorite veggies, fresh herbs, or sprouts for flare and flavor.

Ingredients

1 cup quinoa (traditional or red Incan)

2 cups water

1 cup broccoli florets

1 carrot, sliced diagonally

½ red bell pepper, sliced

2 heads bok choy, quartered

To prepare quinoa:

Put quinoa and water in 1½-quart saucepan, and bring to boil. Reduce heat to simmer; cover and let cook until all water is absorbed (10-15 minutes). When done, the grain appears translucent and the germ ring will be visible. Makes 4 cups.

To prepare bowl:

Gently steam vegetables or blanch in hot water for 30 seconds. Do not overcook as you want them crunchy and to retain as much of their enzymes as possible.

Assemble by placing the quinoa in a serving bowl, top with vegetables, and drizzle with Teriyaki Sauce. Serving size may vary by increasing vegetables and sauce recipe.

Teriyaki Sauce

Ingredients

½ cup Nama Shoyu or tamari

½ cup raw wild honey

red pepper flakes (optional)

Directions

Heat Nama Shoyu and honey together in saucepan, or mix by hand in a bowl, uncooked, for the raw version. The remaining sauce will keep in an airtight container in the refrigerator for up to 1 month.

Nama Shoyu is full of health-giving live enzymes.

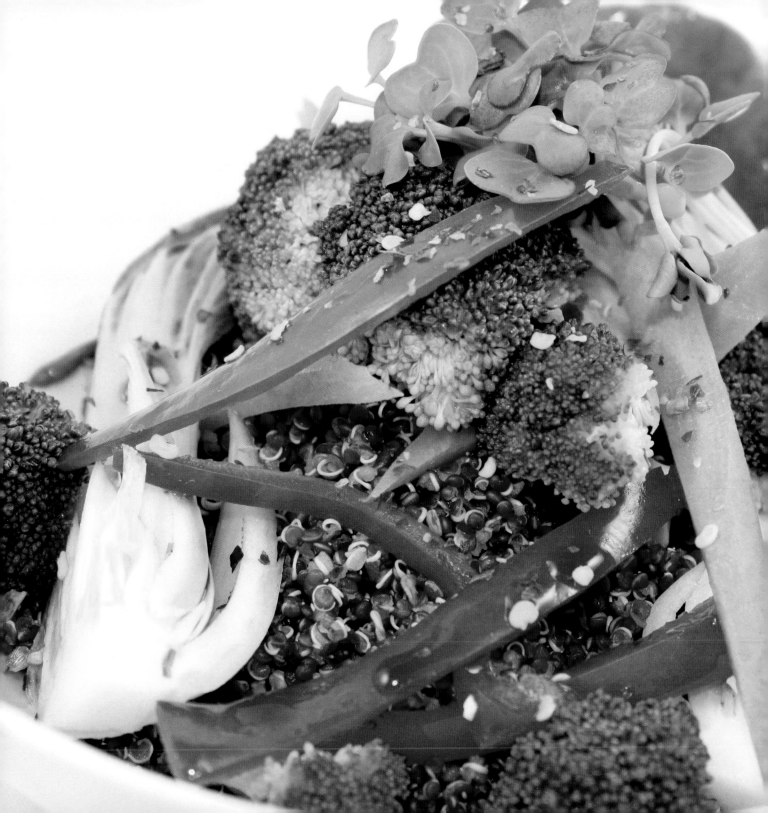

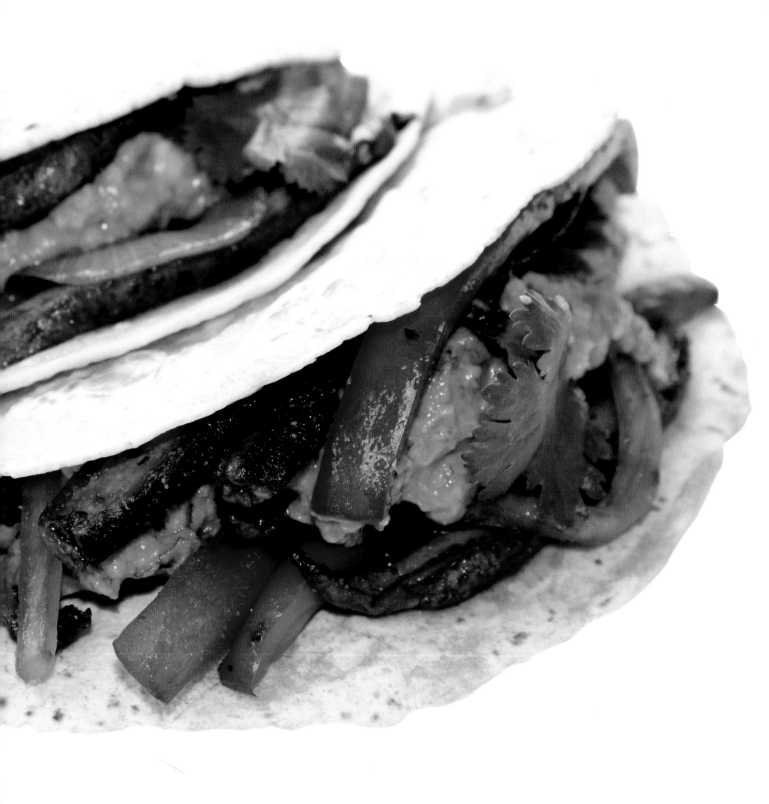

Portobello Mushroom Fajitas

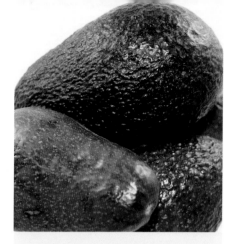

Makes 4-6 servings • Prep time: 20-25 minutes

When I developed this recipe, I had no idea what a monster I was creating—it was such a hit with my family that I'm asked to make it every other day. They love it every time!

Ingredients

4 spelt tortillas or sprouted grain tortillas

2 large Portobello mushrooms, sliced

1 red bell pepper, sliced

1 sweet onion, sliced

1 tablespoon Nama Shoyu

1 teaspoon cumin, ground

1 tablespoon ghee

Guacamole

1 tomato, diced

Directions

Marinate vegetables in Nama Shoyu and cumin for 15 minutes. Sauté veggies in ghee for 3-4 minutes. Remove from heat. Warm the tortillas on a flat sauté pan. Fill each tortilla with veggies and guacamole, and top with diced tomatoes.

Guacamole

Ingredients

2 avocados, mashed

¼ yellow onion, finely chopped

¼ cup cilantro, finely chopped

½ jalapeño pepper, finely chopped

1 lime, juiced

½ teaspoon sea salt

Directions

Mash the avocados with a fork. Add onion, cilantro, and jalapeño. Squeeze lime over mixture and sprinkle with salt. Gently fold ingredients together. Adjust for flavor if needed. Makes 2-4 servings.

Spicy Lentil Tostadas

Makes 4 servings • Prep time: 30-40 minutes

Loaded with fiber, protein, and spice, these tostadas are a true treat. Make sure to load lots of Guacamole and lettuce on top to really round out the flavors.

Ingredients

1 cup lentils, rinsed and cleaned

2 cups water

1 Pasilla chile or Poblano, minced

½ yellow onion, minced

½ cup cilantro, minced

1 cup tomatoes, seeded and diced

1 tablespoon ghee

1 cup Pacific Foods organic vegetable broth

1 teaspoon cumin, ground

1 teaspoon coriander, ground

½ teaspoon paprika

1 teaspoon sea salt

½ teaspoon cayenne pepper

Guacamole (page 83)

8 sprouted corn tortillas

2 cups Romaine lettuce, shredded

To prepare the lentils:

In a 2-quart saucepan, bring water to a boil and add lentils. Let boil for an additional 2 minutes, then place lid on top and lower to simmer. Cook for 20 minutes. Do not drain excess water.

To prepare tostada mixture:

In 10-inch sauté pan, sauté chile, onion, cilantro, and tomato in ghee for 3 minutes. Add the lentils, spices, and broth. Let simmer for 8 minutes, stirring occasionally.

To assemble tostada:

To assemble, heat your tortillas in a flat skillet, or toast them for a crunchy shell. Place a scoop of lentils on the tortilla, add a layer of Guacamole, and top with shredded lettuce. Garnish with fresh cilantro.

. . . .

Lentils are high in protein and loaded with minerals.

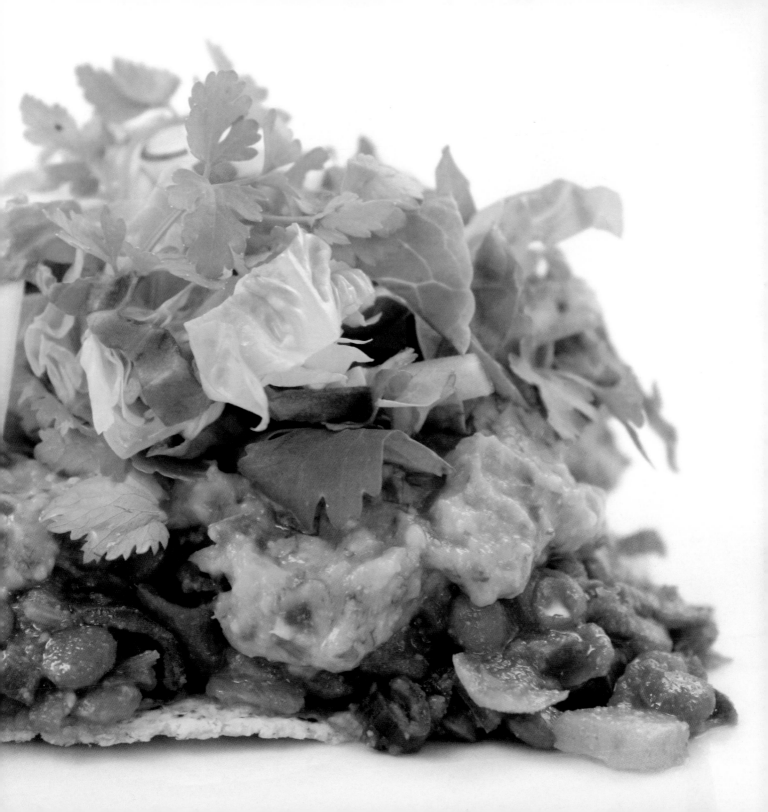

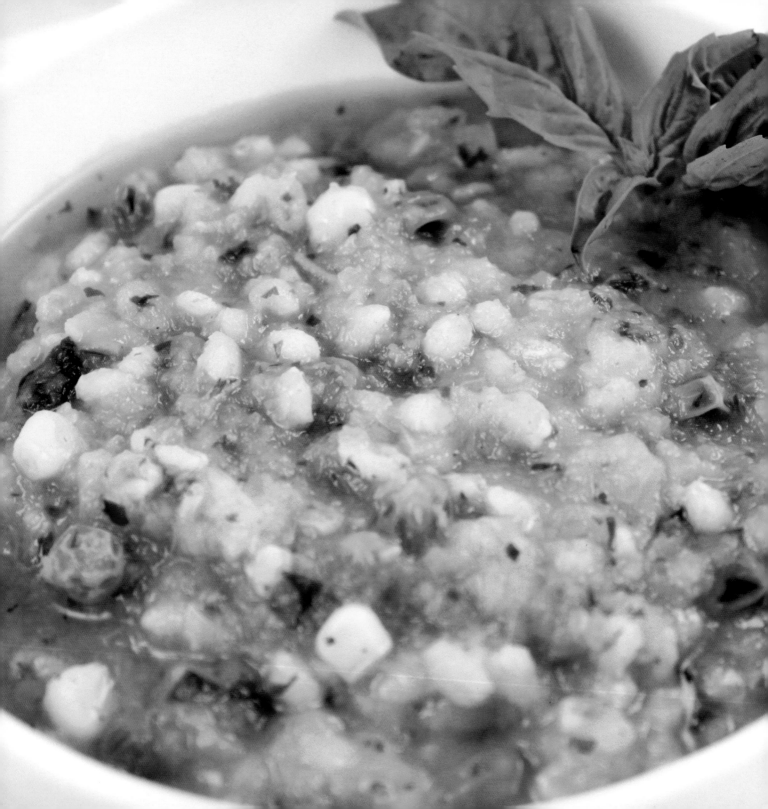

Barley Stew

Makes 4 servings • Prep time: 60 minutes

I have made this stew two ways: one blended for thickness and the other chunky and soupy. The recipe calls for blending, but go for soupy if you prefer one less step. Either way, it's a savory offering of nutrients.

Ingredients

2 tablespoons ghee

2 carrots, diced

1 head of green cabbage, shredded

1 onion, diced

3 stalks celery, diced

1 bunch of basil leaves

2 quarts Pacific Foods organic vegetable broth

1½ teaspoons sea salt

1 cup organic pearl barley

1 cup frozen organic peas

1 cup frozen organic corn

Chopped fresh herbs for garnish (optional)

Directions

In 4-quart sauté pan, sauté carrots, cabbage, onion, celery, and basil in ghee. Add vegetable broth and simmer for 15 minutes on medium-low heat until vegetables are tender. Using immersion blender directly in pot, blend to create a soupy puree. If you do not own an immersion blender, turn heat off and cool stew to room temperature. Use slotted spoon to transfer vegetables to blender, adding just enough broth to blend into a creamy consistency. Pour blended vegetables back into pot with remaining liquid. Add sea salt, peas, corn, barley, and simmer for an additional 30-40 minutes, until barley is cooked. Adjust seasoning if necessary.

Raw Marinated Mushroom Steaks

with Rosemary Mashed Cauliflower

Makes 4 servings • Prep time: 30 minutes

This is a true raw meal, and the mashed cauliflower is going to blow your mind with its rich and creamy taste. Don't be alarmed if you can't eat it all—your body does not need a lot of food when you're eating a raw diet.

Ingredients

4 Portobello mushrooms, washed, stem and gills removed

¼ cup olive oil

1 tablespoon Ume vinegar

1 teaspoon Nama Shoyu

½ teaspoon garlic, freshly grated

Directions

Fold ingredients together in bowl or resealable plastic bag. Let marinate at room temperature for 15 minutes, tossing and basting every few minutes. Reserve extra marinade.

To serve:

Mound Rosemary Mashed Cauliflower onto serving plate, lay portobello steak over top and drizzle with reserved marinade. Garnish each serving with a fresh sprig of rosemary.

*If you would prefer a cooked version of this recipe, gently grill the mushroom steaks.

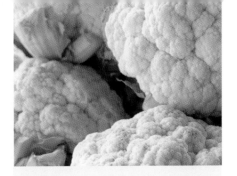

Rosemary Mashed Cauliflower

Ingredients

1 head cauliflower, chopped or broken into florets

½ cup macadamia nut butter

2 tablespoons olive oil

1 teaspoon fresh rosemary, minced

½ teaspoon garlic, peeled and grated

½ teaspoon sea salt

4 sprigs rosemary for garnish (optional)

Directions

Lightly steam cauliflower, or blanch in hot water for 3-5 minutes. Drain and place in processor fitted with an s-blade. Process the cauliflower until it is grainy or reaches the texture of rice. Add macadamia butter, olive oil, herbs, and spices and process until light and fluffy, scraping sides frequently. This could take up to 5 minutes for desired consistency.

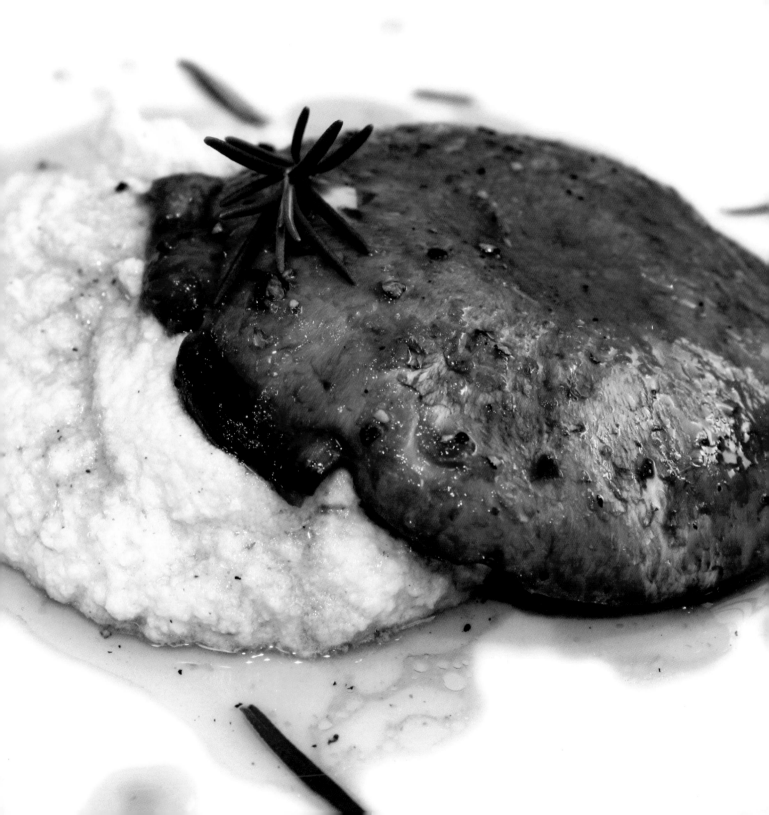

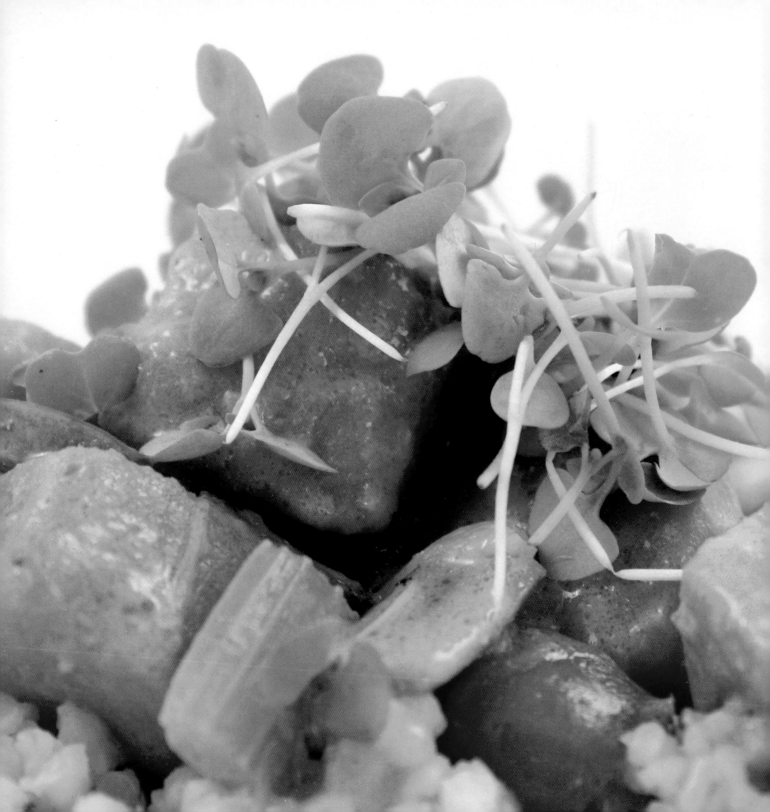

Sweet Potato Curry

Makes 4 servings • Prep time: 40-45 minutes

I like a sweet creamy curry, and this dish is exactly that. The sweet potatoes mixed with the Fresh Coconut Milk and spices are a treat for the delicate palate. Canned coconut milk is not preferable, as canned foods are acidic, but it does work in a pinch.

Curry

1 large sweet potato, peeled, cut into 1-inch chunks

1 medium onion, diced into 1-inch chunks

2 stalks celery, sliced into 1-inch chunks

1 large carrot, sliced into 1-inch chunks

1 red bell pepper, diced into 1-inch chunks

1 tablespoon ghee

3 cups Fresh Coconut Milk (page 92)

1 tablespoon turmeric

2 teaspoons garam masala

1 teaspoon cumin, ground

1 teaspoon sea salt

½ teaspoon black pepper, freshly ground

Fresh cilantro leaves (for garnish)

Rice

1 cup organic short or long grain brown rice

1¾ cups water

½ teaspoon sea salt

Place all ingredients in a 1½-quart saucepan, heat on high until it reaches a boil. Lower to simmer and cook, covered, for 35 minutes. Remove from heat, let sit for a few minutes, and then serve.

To prepare curry:

In 3-quart saucepan on medium heat, sauté vegetables in ghee for 2-3 minutes. Add turmeric, garam masala, cumin, salt, pepper, and Fresh Coconut Milk. Simmer about 10 minutes, or until vegetables are desired texture. Pour over rice and garnish with fresh cilantro.

It is important to cut vegetables to a consistent size.
They look more appealing and will cook evenly for a better distribution of flavor.

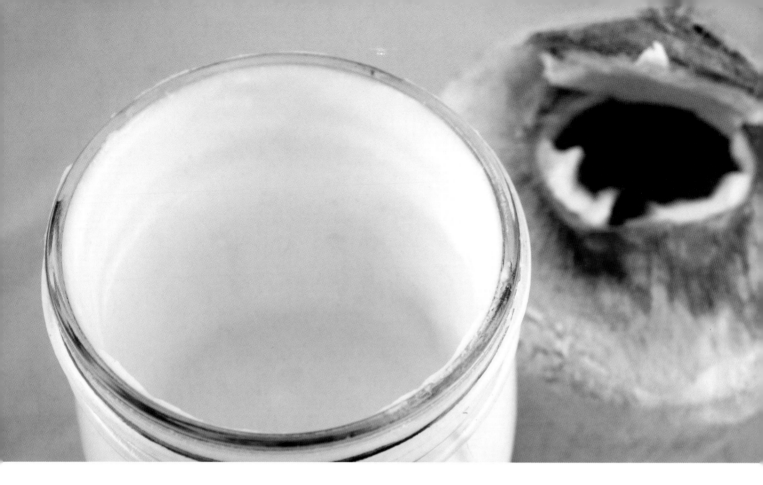

Fresh Coconut Milk

Makes 3 cups

(You may need 2 coconuts)

1½ cups coconut meat

1½ cups coconut water

Blend coconut meat and coconut water in high-speed blender until smooth and creamy.

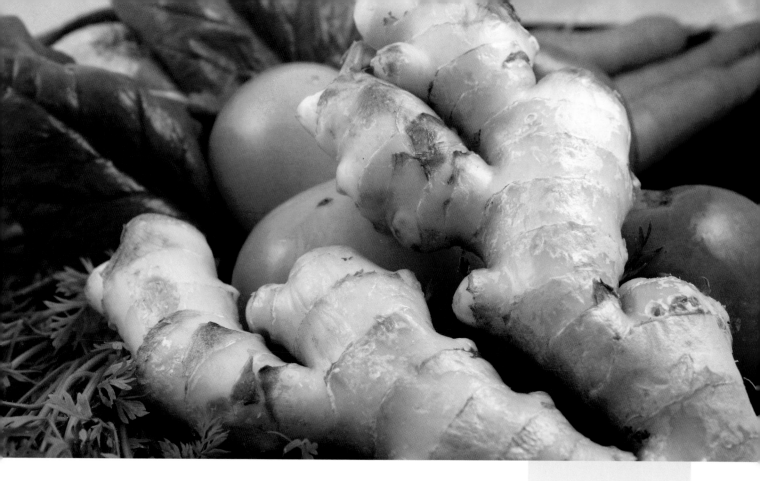

Foods That Nourish the Kidneys

- Barley
- Quinoa
- Wheat Berries
- Adzuki Beans
- Black Beans
- Kidney Beans
- Fennel

- Onions
- Spring Onions
- Chives
- Black Sesame Seeds
- Beetroot
- Parsley
- Celery

- Blackberries
- Blueberries
- Mung Beans
- Walnuts
- Seaweed
- Chlorella

Teas/Herbs

- Cloves
- Cinnamon Bark
- Fenugreek
- Garlic
- Ginger
- Raspberry
- Blackberry
- Rose hips
- Dandelion

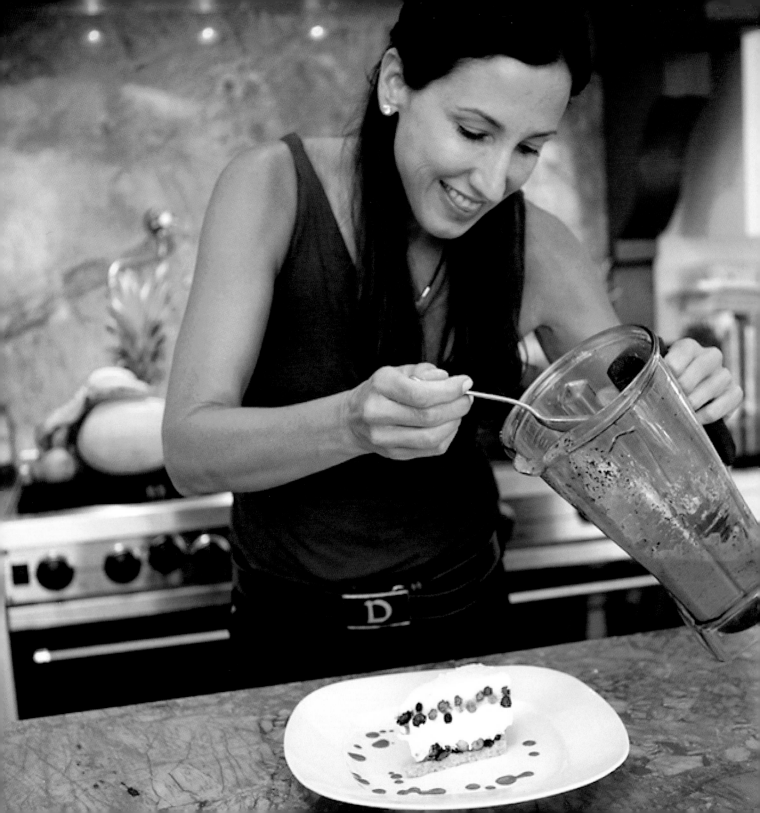

Satisfying Sweets

Sometimes it's just nice to nibble on something sweet.
The beauty of Naked foods is that we have delicious,
natural choices that are not only suitable to your palate,
but satisfying as well. There is always room for plain fruit,
and there really is nothing better than fresh fruit in season.
With this in mind, it's best to stick with low glycemic
foods in the evening so you're able to sleep. For example,
berries and citrus are good choices, but watermelon
is not because its sugar content excites the system.
These dessert recipes make a great snack any time of
the day when you are craving something sweet, and are
impressive when entertaining guests.

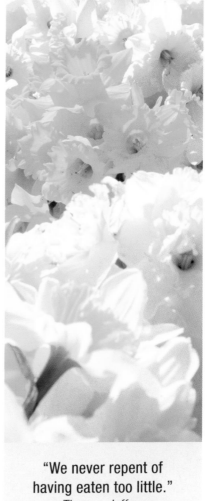

**"We never repent of
having eaten too little."**
~ *Thomas Jefferson*

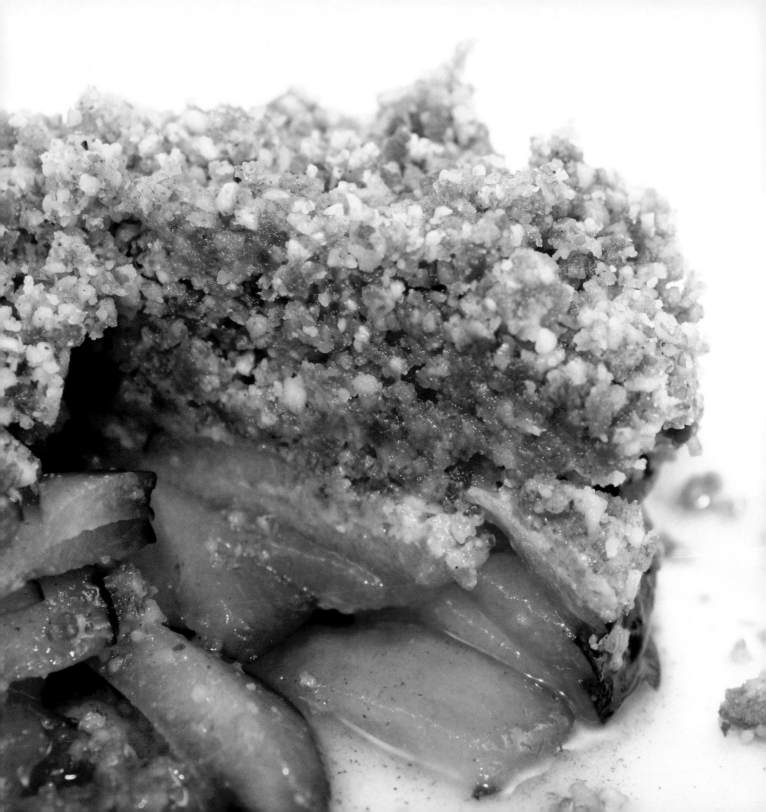

Plum Crisp

Makes 1 serving • Prep time: 10 minutes

Prepare this in a tart mold for an elegant-looking dessert. Each plum has its own unique flavor, so this recipe tastes unique and spectacular every time. Other fruits, such as peaches, berries, or apples may be substituted.

Ingredients

- 2 plums, seeded and sliced thin
- ½ teaspoon agave
- ¼ teaspoon cinnamon

Directions

Toss sliced plums, agave, and cinnamon together in bowl and let sit to infuse flavors while preparing topping.

Crisp

Ingredients

- ¼ cup raw pecans
- 1 Medjool date, pitted and chopped
- 1/8 teaspoon cinnamon
- 1/8 teaspoon vanilla powder
- 1/8 teaspoon sea salt

Directions

Place all ingredients in processor fitted with s-blade. Pulse until pecans and dates are broken down. Place sliced plums in serving dish of choice. Crumble pecan-date mixture on top of plums, then press lightly to form a crusty top. Enjoy as is or serve with your favorite non-dairy frozen dessert.

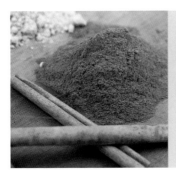

 FUN FACT: Cinnamon is the bark of a small tree and is one of the world's oldest spices.

 NUTRITIONAL BENEFIT: Cinnamon is a supreme digestive tonic.

 HOW TO SELECT: Select organic, as possible, freshly grind just prior to use.

Mango Sorbet

Makes 1 serving • Prep time: 7 minutes

Who knew a light and refreshing dessert could be this easy? Garnish with Blueberries for a color burst and an antioxidant boost.

Ingredients

    1 cup frozen organic mango chunks

Directions

Allow mango chunks to defrost for 5 minutes in processor fitted with s-blade. Process until smooth. Serve immediately.

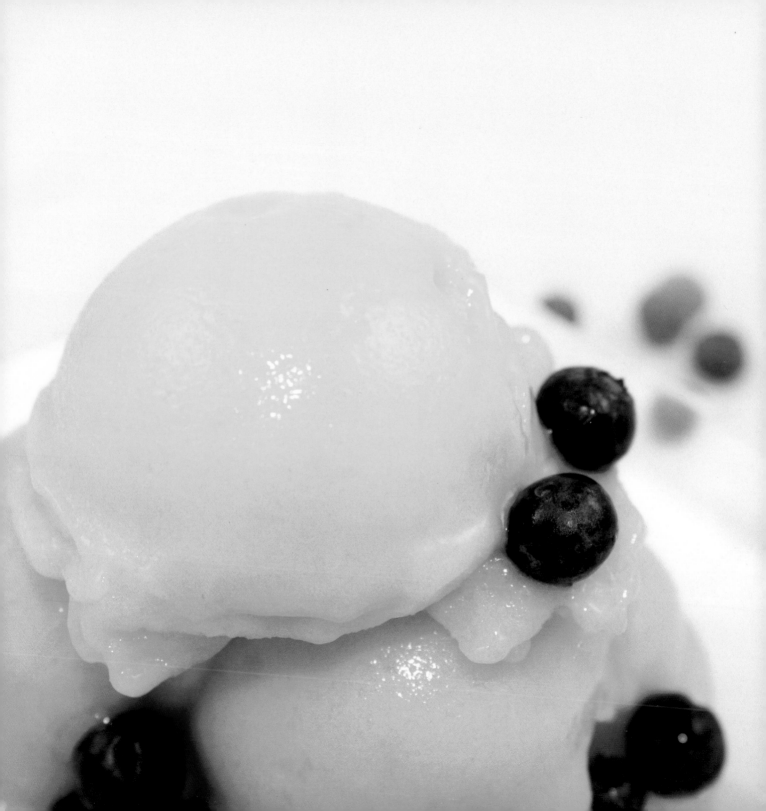

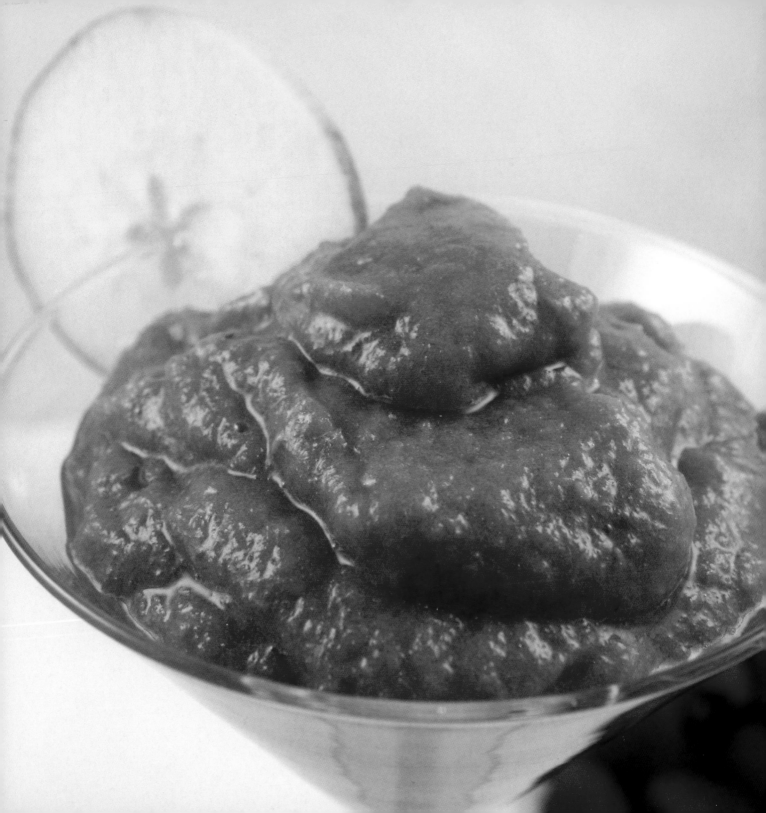

Raspberry Applesauce

Makes 1 serving • Prep time: 5 minutes

Color, texture, and flavor—oh my! For an icier version, substitute organic frozen raspberries for fresh.

Ingredients

1 apple, cored, peeled, and chopped

1 pint raspberries

2 Medjool dates, pitted

Directions

Place all ingredients in processor or blender. Process until smooth.

Raspberries are packed with powerful antioxidants and vitamin C, which is great for glowing skin.

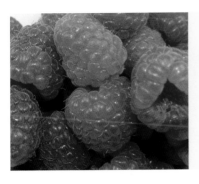

 FUN FACT: Raspberries are part of the genus *Rubus,* which is a member of the Rose family.

 NUTRITIONAL BENEFIT: Raspberries are high with vitamin C and considered a tonic for kidneys and liver.

 HOW TO SELECT: Choose berries that feel dry to the touch and have hollow centers.

Walnut-Pecan Brownies

Makes 6 brownies • Prep time: less than 10 minutes

One taste of these delicious brownies, and you will never crave another sugar-laden version again. Be careful not to overprocess, as the oils will begin to release and you'll end up with a sticky brownie.

Ingredients
½ cup raw walnuts

½ cup raw pecans

¼ cup raw cacao powder

½ cup Medjool dates, pitted and firmly packed

Directions
Place walnuts and pecans in processor fitted with s-blade and pulse until nuts are a finely ground. Add dates and cacao and process until mixture begins to stick together. Do not over process. Place mixture into a 4x9 loaf pan lined with parchment paper, garnish with pecans and slice into 6 squares. Or, use a square cookie cutter and form individual servings by dividing mixture into 6 portions and pressing firmly into the cookie mold. Gently remove the mold and garnish with chopped pecans.

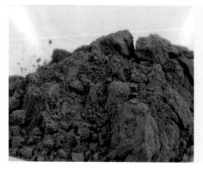

 FUN FACT: Raw cacao matches the brain chemicals we have when excited, happy or sexually aroused.

 NUTRITIONAL BENEFIT: Cacao is high in flavonoids which and helps promote cardio-vascular health.

 HOW TO SELECT: Select raw cacao not cocoa powder.

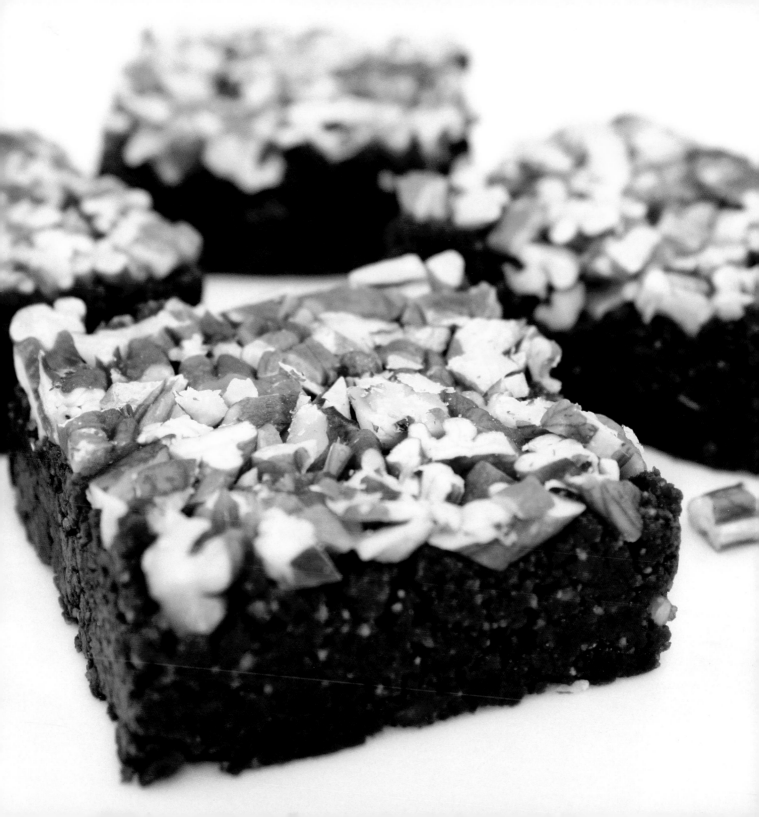

Pecan-Pie Treats

Makes 1 serving • Prep time: none

*I have such a sweet tooth, and these were a staple in my diet when I first began my transition to raw.
An excellent treat to satisfy your sweet cravings, you can eat them like a cookie!*

Ingredients
2-3 Medjool dates

4-6 raw pecan halves

Directions
Slice dates in half and remove pit. Press pecan halves into soft spots of dates, similar to making a sandwich.

Dates contain 31 grams of carbohydrates, making them a powerhouse of energy.

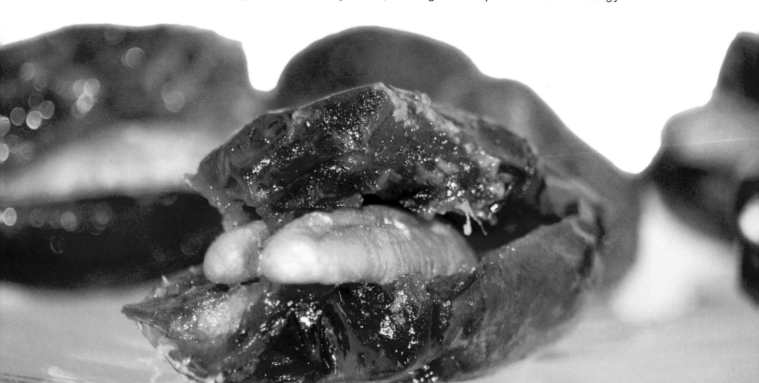

Spiced Bananas

Makes 1 serving • Prep time: less than 5 minutes

Flavorful and high in minerals, these lovely bathed bananas pair nicely with a non-dairy frozen dessert. Try substituting cloves or cinnamon for a different flavor.

Ingredients

- 1 banana, sliced
- ¼ cup orange juice, freshly squeezed
- 1 teaspoon raw honey
- 1/8 teaspoon star anise, ground or powdered
- Orange zest

Directions

Whisk together orange juice, honey and star anise, and pour over banana slices. Garnish with orange zest.

Citrus is not only high in vitamin C, but it has also been said to suppress appetites.

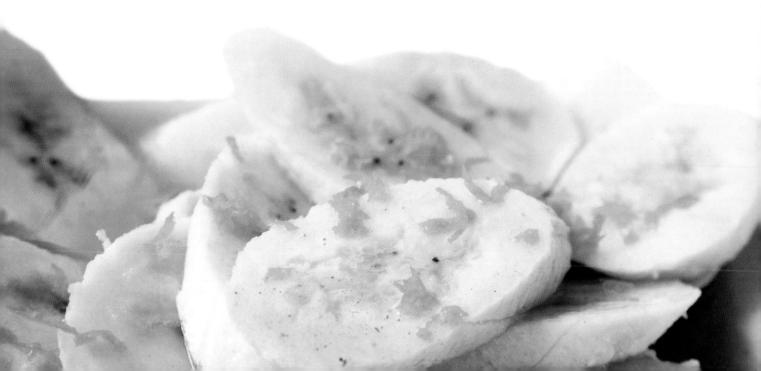

Chocolate Fondue

Makes 2 servings • Prep time: less than 5 minutes

Every fruit is enjoyable with chocolate, so try this with fresh organic kiwi, bananas, raspberries—whatever you like. Sometimes I just like to dip my fingers in this luscious treat.

Ingredients

¼ cup raw cacao powder

¼ cup agave nectar

1 teaspoon vanilla extract

2 tablespoons coconut oil

Directions

Place the coconut oil jar in a hot bath to soften the oil. Combine cacao, agave, and vanilla in small mixing bowl. Add melted coconut oil and whisk together until creamy. Place fruit on the tip of bamboo skewers and begin dipping. Fondue may be stored in an airtight container, at room temperature, for up to 1 month.

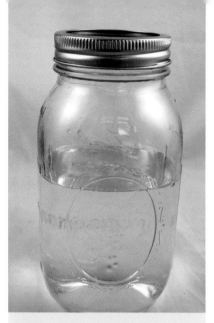

 FUN FACT: Coconut oil is highly moisturizing and promotes elasticity in the skin.

NUTRITIONAL BENEFIT: Coconut oil increases metabolism and helps the body break up accumulated fat.

 HOW TO SELECT: Raw virgin coconut oil

Cacao has been said to create an uncontrollable state of bliss.

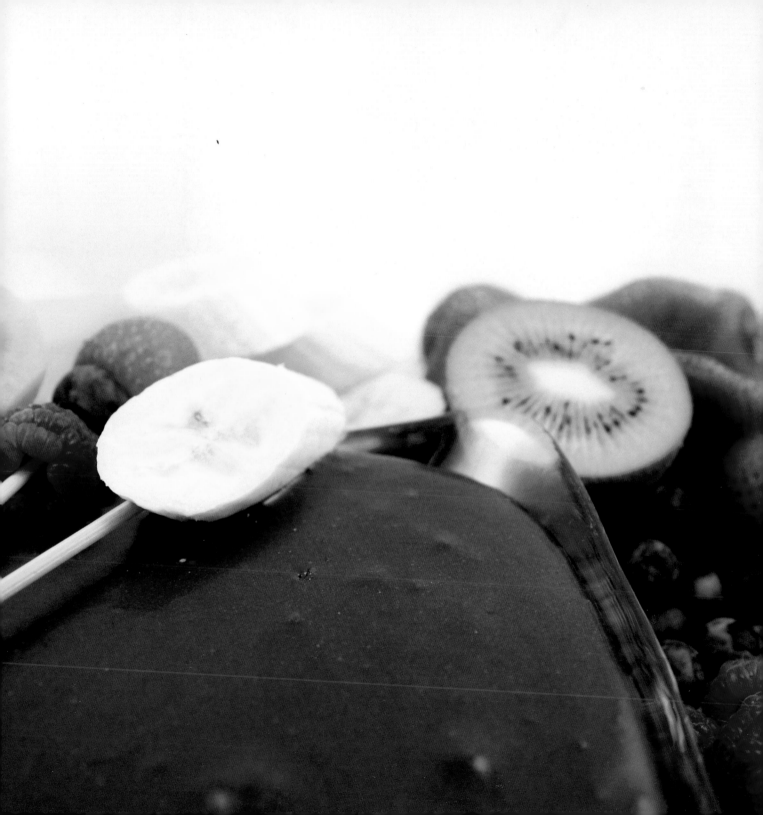

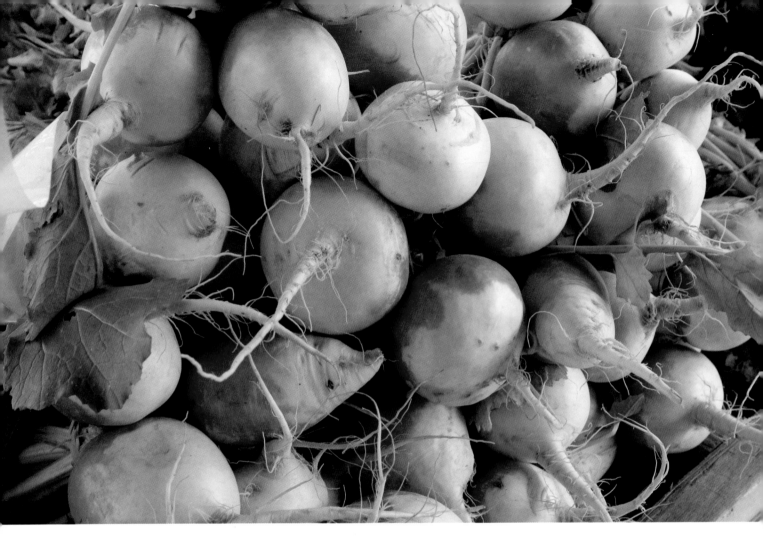

Foods That Nourish the Liver

- Broccoli
- Brussels Sprouts
- Cabbage
- Cauliflower

- Garlic
- Kohlrabi
- Turnip Roots
- Nuts

- Flax Seeds
- Sunflower Seeds
- Pumpkin Seeds

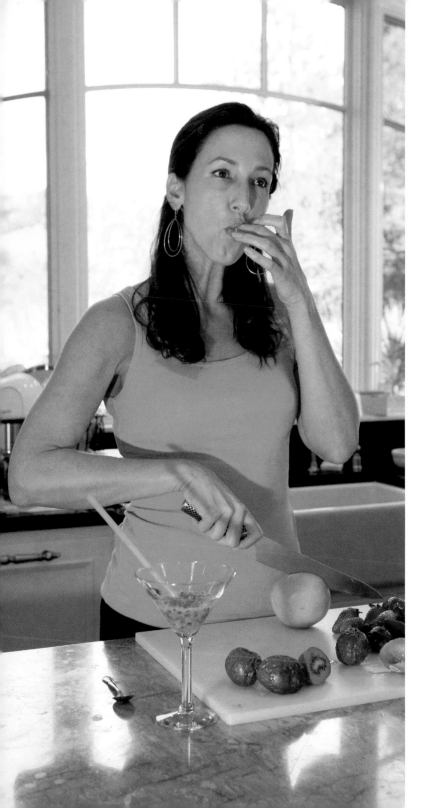

Beauty Elixirs

These beautifying recipes can serve as both a thirst quencher and a snack. At any time during the day, go for a drink if you would like a delicious, nutritious pick-me-up. It will not only hydrate you, but also give you an instant energy boost. I consider these drinks a full meal, as they are extremely satisfying; I don't typically pair them with another meal because it would be too much food. The blended drinks are particularly uplifting since a high-speed blender breaks down the ingredients to such a degree that your body can easily assimilate the energy and nutrients from the live produce. Please remember to drink a lot of water as well; water is a purifier and has a natural cleansing effect on the body.

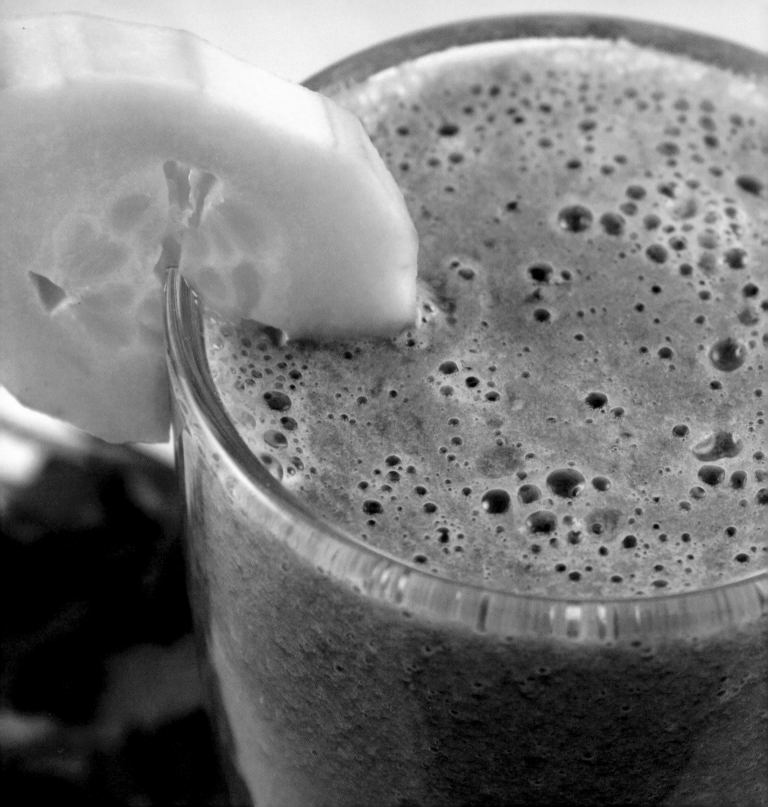

Extra Virgin Bloody Mary

Makes 2 servings • Prep time: less than 5 minutes

Reminiscent of the classic cocktail, this is a wonderful cleansing treat on your palate and for your body.

Ingredients

2 large tomatoes

1/2 cucumber

1 stalk celery

1/2 cup spinach

1/4 cup parsley

2 tablespoons yellow onion, diced

1 cup purified water

2 tablespoons lemon juice, freshly squeezed

1/2 teaspoon sea salt, or to taste

pinch cayenne pepper

Directions

Place all ingredients in high-speed blender and blend until smooth. If you like a smoother drink without the pulp, strain through a nut milk bag or fine mesh strainer. Will last up to 2 days refrigerated.

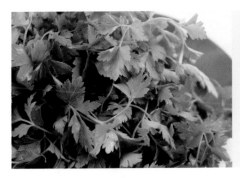

 FUN FACT: Parsley is high in chlorophyll and freshens breath.

 NUTRITIONAL BENEFIT: Parsley is used as a remedy for arthritis and edema.

 HOW TO SELECT: Look for parsley that is deep green in color.

Kiwi Lemonade

Serves 1 • Prep time: less than 5 minutes

This is an amazing and tart combination. Kiwis vary in sweetness, so adjust the agave accordingly.

Kiwis are loaded with vitamin C.

Ingredients

1 lemon, freshly squeezed

1 kiwi, peeled and sliced

1-2 tablespoons agave nectar (as desired)

2 cups water

Directions

Reserve one kiwi slice for garnish. Place all other ingredients in blender. Blend on high for 60 seconds, pour over ice, and add garnish. Additional ice may be added to blender for a slushier version.

To ripen firm kiwis, place them at room temperature away from heat and sunlight for a few days.

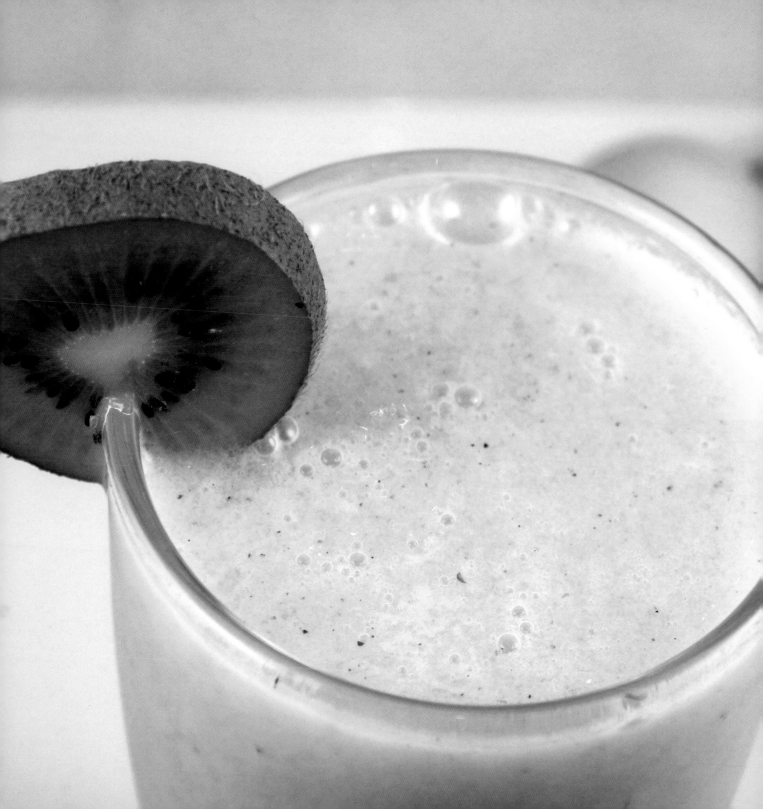

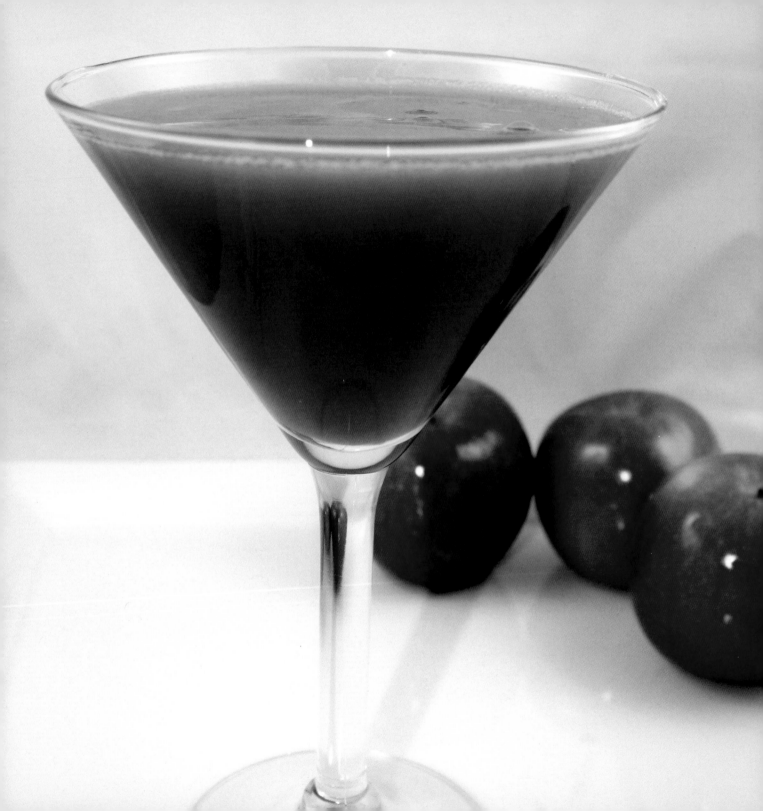

Green Appletini

Makes 1 serving • Prep time: less than 5 minutes

Half the fun of cocktail hour is holding beautiful stemware, sipping an exotic drink, and having conversation. This "rawktail" will keep you in the mix as well as healthy and happy. Serve in a martini glass for flare and pizzazz!

Ingredients

1 1/2 cups water

1 large Fuji apple (or other sweet apple of choice), cored and sliced

1 cup fresh baby spinach

3 tablespoons lemon juice, freshly squeezed

2 tablespoons agave nectar

Directions

Blend all ingredients in high-speed blender until smooth. Strain through a fine sieve or nut-milk bag for a pulp-free "rawktail," or enjoy its natural pulp straight up.

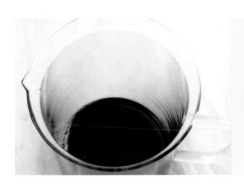

 FUN FACT: American natives revered the agave plant as sacred, purifying the body and soul.

 NUTRITIONAL BENEFIT: Agave is a low glycemic sweetener.

 HOW TO SELECT: Choose light agave nectar.

Orange Magic

Makes 1 serving • Prep time: less than 5 minutes

This drink is a meal in itself—it's like drinking a salad! Red leaf lettuce and mache greens are my favorite to use in this recipe.

Ingredients

1½ cups orange juice, freshly squeezed (approximately 2-3 oranges)

½ cucumber, peeled and sliced

1 cup salad greens

1 tablespoon flaxseed oil, or Udo's Choice™ Oil Blend

Directions

Place freshly squeezed orange juice, sliced cucumber, and favorite salad greens with oil into high-speed blender.

Blend on high for 60 seconds, then serve. If a smoother consistency is desired, strain through a fine mesh strainer.

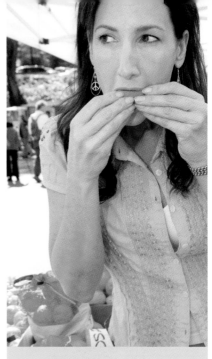

Oranges are high in vitamin C and fiber.

Citrus and greens create magic in your body: they are alkaline and very cleansing.

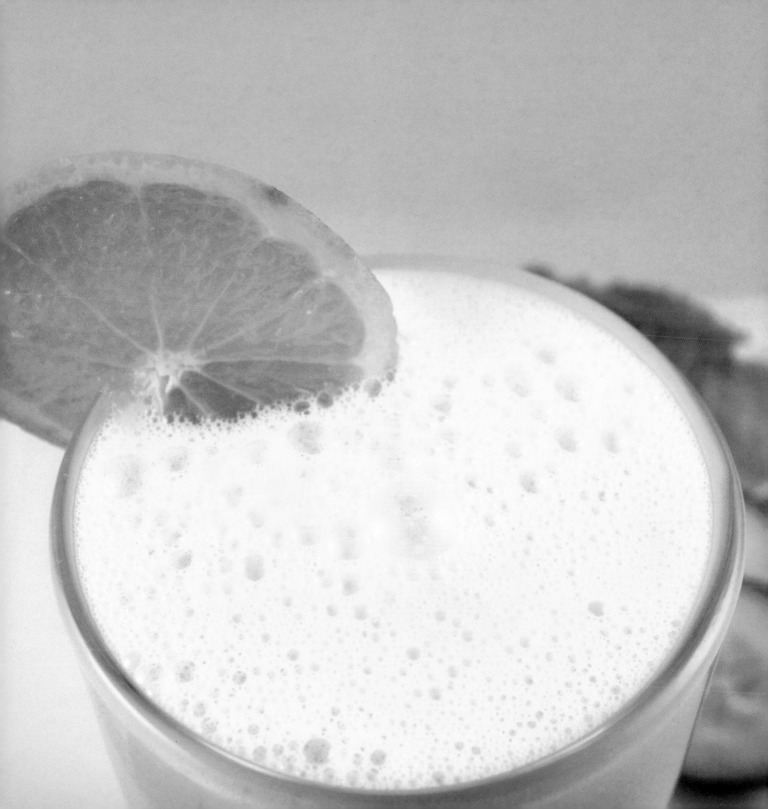

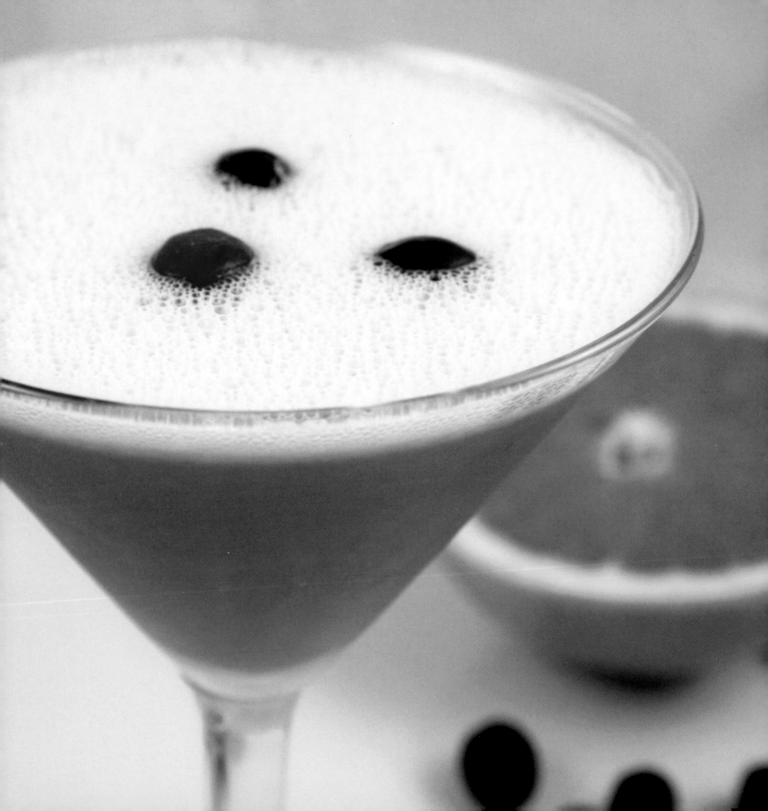

Pink Grapefruit Cosmopolitan

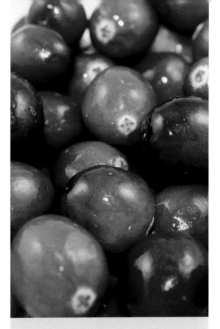

Cranberries are cleansing
for both the liver
and kidneys.

Makes 1 serving • Prep time: less than 5 minutes

When it's cocktail time and you want something refreshing and beautifying, this is the perfect choice.

Ingredients

   1 grapefruit, freshly squeezed

   5 cranberries, fresh or frozen (extra for garnishing)

   1-2 teaspoons agave nectar (as desired)

   1 handful of ice

Directions

Place grapefruit juice, cranberries, agave nectar, and ice in blender and blend on high for 60 seconds. Pour mixture through fine mesh strainer into martini glass. Garnish with a cranberry.

Drinking astringent fruits like grapefruit and cranberries will get the
lymph nodes moving and flush the body of cellulite.

Coconut Dream

Makes 1 serving • Prep time: 2 minutes

Nothing is more hydrating and satisfying! Add mint, lemon, or raspberries for a flavored coconut water treat.

Ingredients
  1 young Thai Coconut

Directions
Crack open coconut and sip through a straw. Alternatively, pour coconut water in blender with meat and blend for a creamier version. Add ice for a cool, slushy version.

Cracking open a young Thai coconut is an experience in itself. Another option is to have your local Asian market or health food store produce manager open it for you.

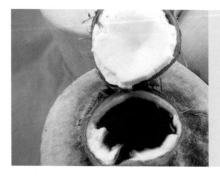

 FUN FACT: Coconut water is considered the fluid of life, as it has been used to replace blood plasma.

 NUTRITIONAL BENEFIT: Coconut water is a natural isotonic beverage as it contains the perfect electrolyte balance.

 HOW TO SELECT: Look for clear, transparent liquid, not purplish.

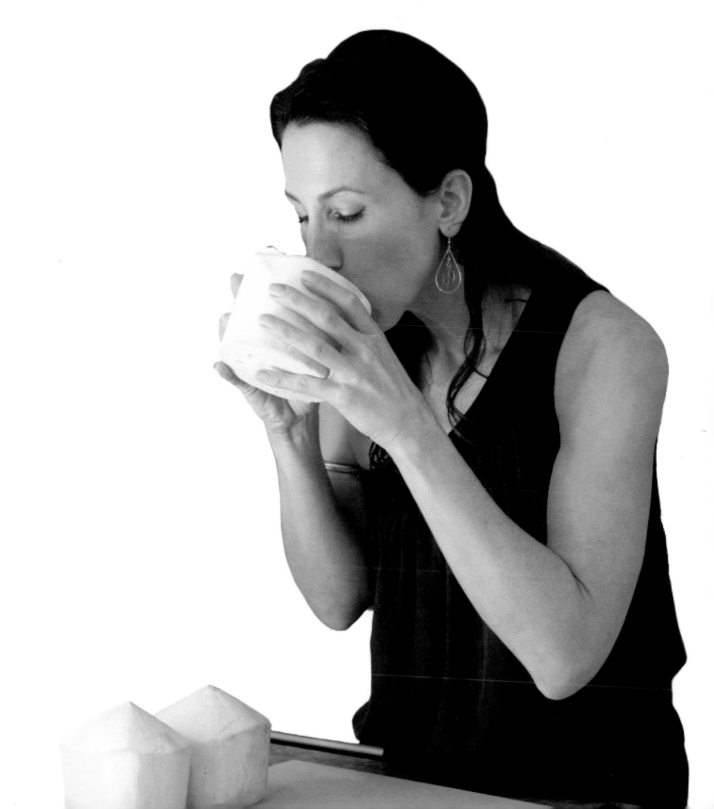

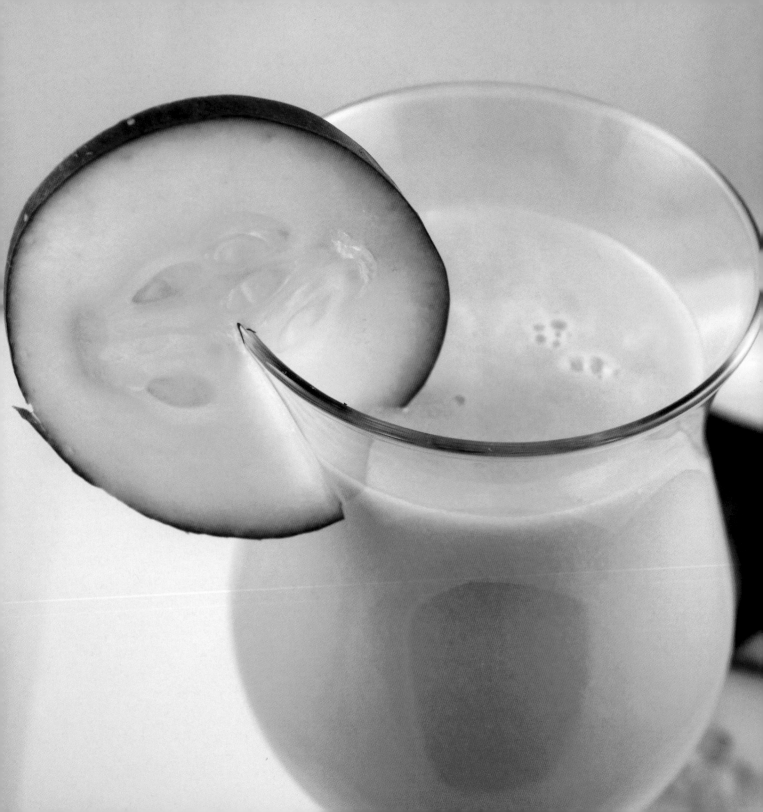

Melon Smoothie

Makes 1 serving • Prep time: less than 5 minutes

Packed with vitamin C and potassium, this is a delicious and tasty drink. The cucumber adds hydration, and the oil lubricates the organs and makes for a frothier drink. You may peel the cucumber if you prefer less pulp, but keep in mind most of the nutrients are in the skin.

Ingredients

½ cantaloupe or honeydew, diced
(approximately 2 cups)

½ cucumber, diced

1 tablespoon flaxseed oil or Udo's Choice™ Oil Blend (optional)

Directions

Place melon and cucumber in blender and blend on high for 60 seconds. Add a small amount of water, if necessary, to get your blender working.

Foods That Nourish Your Body Naked!

Extra Beautifying Foods, Extra Sexy Foods

- Apples
- Artichokes
- Asparagus
- Avocados
- Bananas
- Beetroot
- Blackberries
- Blackcurrants
- Blueberries
- Brazil Nuts
- Brown Rice
- Cardamom
- Celery

- Cherries
- Chia Seeds
- Chives
- Chlorella
- Cinnamon
- Daikon Radishes
- Dates
- Dulse Seaweed
- Fennel
- Figs
- Flax Seeds
- Garlic
- Ginger
- Goldenberries
- Hazelnuts

- Leeks
- Licorice
- Mangos
- Mung Beans
- Nori Seaweed
- Nutmeg
- Oats
- Okra
- Onions
- Parsley
- Pomegranates
- Pumpkins
- Pumpkin Seeds
- Quinoa
- Raspberries

- Raw Sauerkraut
- Saffron
- Seaweed
- Sesame Seeds
- Soaked Almonds
- Spinach
- Spirulina
- Squash Seeds
- Kale
- Strawberries
- Sunflower Seeds
- Tomatoes
- Turmeric
- Vanilla
- Watercress

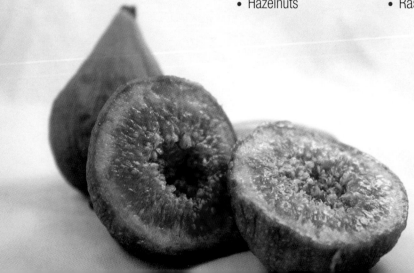

Diana's Walk-Away Message

I began writing this book with the intention of providing a quick guide to get people started toward good health. As I began to put together various bits of material, I suddenly realized that my real intention was not to provide a quick fix for health, but to lay a stepping stone for the path to wellness. I realize there are unexpected twists and turns along this wonderful path of life, and every day is a new opportunity to make different choices depending on our moods, energy, or state of being. The journey to health is one of the greatest adventures you will ever embark on— it goes beyond the physical and into every aspect of your life. My true love has always been the process of helping people open doors to their own truth, and watching the transformations. Over the years, it is the very thing that motivates me to strive for more and continue creating.

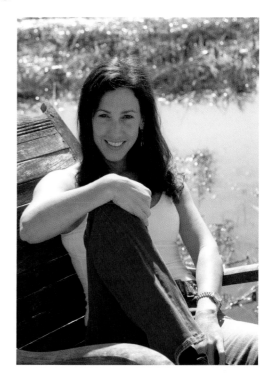

When I envision the potential for optimum health across the world, and the undiscovered energy and youth we all want for ourselves, I smile knowing you have opened your mind and heart to your full potential. I find joy in knowing that if you have indeed followed the steps to getting Naked, that then you are feeling lighter, brighter, and more amazing than ever before. I know you are completely blown away by your good health, beautiful skin, and sexy body that has been transforming before your eyes over the past few weeks. I want to encourage you to keep moving in this positive direction and never look back!

I will constantly be laying new stepping stones of information. I will continue creating and sharing new ways of preparing fun dishes that taste great and keep you alive and vibrant, if you promise to keep eating the foods that nourish you. I thank you for trusting me with your nourishment, and I wholeheartedly congratulate you for taking care of yourself!

-Diana
Because it feels so good!

Recipe Index

About the Author

Culinary artist and raw food enthusiast Diana Stobo is living proof that her Naked Nourishment lifestyle works. Once plagued by relentless pain and physical discomfort due to food toxicity, Diana successfully navigated her way through old patterns to discover a healthy way of eating and living. She has transformed her own life to one of optimum health, vibrance, and beauty. Passionate about everything in life including her relationships, her family, her wellness, and especially her food, Diana understands how integral food is to all aspects of nutrition including child development, family patterns, social expectations, and body awareness.

As someone who looks and feels younger than she did 10 years ago, Diana's philosophy is to empower the individual with food choices that create a better lifestyle. Diana's goal is to design nutritious, accessible products—familiar foods with taste and flare—while introducing exciting and healthful new ingredients. Diana integrates the whole of her experience—from her early teenage tart-baking business, to training in Cornell University's School of Hotel Administration culinary arts division, to running her highly successful Signature Catering business, to consulting one-on-one with clients to tailor individualized programs, to developing a raw snack line for the "tween" pangs of hunger—to emerge in the living food movement as a leading innovator and educator.

Combining professional expertise with rich personal experience, Diana is dedicated to creating delicious, nutritious recipes that are easy to prepare and satisfying to the senses. Feasting while dropping excess weight, increasing physical and mental energy, and staying young and sexy while developing a healthier relationship with food—this is the Naked Nourishment lifestyle that Diana has discovered for herself and wishes to share with you!